DIALOGUE WITH SAMMY

A Psycho-Analytical Contribution to the Understanding of Child Psychosis

Joyce McDougall *and* Serge Lebovici

The story of Sammy, a 10-year-old American boy, whose struggle to convey the content and feeling of his psychotic inner world, forms the heart of this moving book. Driven by overwhelming anxiety, but also impelled by the human need for creation and self-expression, Sammy demanded that his analyst write down verbatim his fantasies and stories. Thus, in a sense, he is the prime author, providing the core material which stimulated Joyce McDougall and Serge Lebovici, two of France's leading child analysts, to add the rich dimensions that a full account of a child analysis and related commentaries could bring. In following the detailed account of the psycho-analytic sessions, the reader can come to feel himself something of the quest together of child and analyst for understanding, in the continually unfolding human drama that is a child analysis. He will admire and wonder at the tact, skill, warmth, and courage that are required of the analyst, and gain some appreciation of the value of psycho-analysis as a therapeutic and research tool in that as yet poorly known world of child psychosis. Yet, if one can yield to a fuller empathy, does not one find something of Sammy in each of us, and does not v_____ throw light on and open to _____ of every man's existence?

DIALOGUE WITH
SAMMY

DIALOGUE WITH SAMMY

*A Psycho-Analytical Contribution to
the Understanding of Child Psychosis*

JOYCE McDOUGALL
AND
SERGE LEBOVICI

Edited by
MARTIN JAMES

11029

NEW YORK
INTERNATIONAL UNIVERSITIES PRESS
1969

This book is an edited translation of
Un Cas de Psychose infantile
Published in 1960 by
Presses Universitaires de France.
It has been revised and translated
from the French by Joyce McDougall

Printed in Great Britain by
R. and R. Clark Ltd
Edinburgh

CONTENTS

Acknowledgements

to Sammy who made this book possible
to Sammy's parents who gave permission to publish it
to the Director of the Special School for his report
finally, to our friend and colleague James Gammill for
his valuable assistance with the English edition

PREFACE

IN the original French version of this book the account of each session is followed by a supervisor's comment, Dr Serge Lebovici being the supervisor. What has been lost in this English edition by the omission of these comments (which the reader can study in the original book) has perhaps been offset by a more consolidated statement of this boy's analysis. Here now is an account of the analysis of a psychotic boy which students can use, the details of which can be discussed along with the theoretical implications. It is logical to have this book in its English form because the analysis was conducted in the English language, the boy being an American, so that in that respect the original book was a translation into French.

There is in this case the exceptional feature that the boy insisted on accurate notes being taken so that the majority of what happened is recorded in the session. Accurate statements of analytic work with children are not too common and this one will be welcomed not only by those who are studying child analysis but also by those who can enjoy a true story or an autobiography. This boy was very ill, displaying psychotic clinical features, and the year's analysis brought about great changes. It seems unlikely that he would have made these changes towards health simply by growing older or through ordinary life experiences.

The reader can watch what the authors call 'the re-establishment of the dialogue' as Sammy gains confidence in the analyst's reliability and understanding and finds a way of both contributing and accepting.

Another important feature is the way in which a book like this puts those of us who principally read English in touch with the work of Lebovici, Diatkine, Bouvet and others, who write almost exclusively in the French language.

Advice can be given to the reader of a book like this; there is something to be gained from a double reading. The first reading could be a quick one free from the effort to make the most of the rich detail of the sessions. Such a quick reading would enable the reader to get the feeling of the sweep of the whole story and to locate the phases in which there was the greatest difficulty which by being resolved brought about the greatest progress. Such a phase would be when Sammy became identified with the wild horse and responsible for the farts; also there was the time when he did actually hurt his analyst and provoked her into a change in technique, all of which proved profitable in the long run.

In the second reading the reader could allow full enjoyment of the details dictated by Sammy and also in all the management problems which the analyst had to meet.

The first story, that of 'Le Visage magique', is itself so full of interest that if one allows oneself to get caught up in it one can fail to reach to a total view of the analysis. In fact one could get stuck at the very beginning where, as is reported, Sammy 'Draws in a curious fashion . . . as though he were feeling round the edges of objects, reproducing what he touches rather than what he sees.' One can say that some patients are lucky when their analysts do not understand too much at the beginning so that they can feel round and have full opportunity for creative impressions. Gradually they like to be understood, but they may feel cheated if understood so quickly that the analyst seems to be a magician.

One feels that in this presentation of an analysis Joyce McDougall's own interpretations have been faithfully given along with the details of her management of the case, and in this way the book with Sammy's own rich contribution, should find a permanent place in the literature of psychotherapy. The authors' comments are enriched by information gained in the subsequent psychotherapy of the boy's mother.

D. W. WINNICOTT

INTRODUCTION

THE story of Sammy's treatment was first published in Paris in 1960. Sammy himself provided the unique opportunity for writing this book: his anxiety in the analytic situation was so great that for many months he would not talk unless Joyce McDougall, his analyst, noted down everything he said. 'Now write what I dictate. I'm your dictator!' he would shout. Sammy was not an easy patient. But the analysis continued, five times a week for the best part of a year, on what Sammy called his 'trouble'. This trouble took manifold shapes. Sammy sometimes located it in the analyst, sometimes in inanimate objects and the world around him. As the analytic work proceeded he began to realise that it was inside himself. His attempts to deal with his trouble frequently sought direct expression in the analytic transference, in a fight against 'Dougie's wicked bosoms' or her dangerous 'knuckle head'; and at other times were expressed through a rich and intricate fantasy world of pathos and, sometimes, of poetic beauty. Later, when Sammy was able to tolerate the anxiety of the analytic situation, he no longer demanded that each word be caught and imprisoned on paper. Thereafter, brief notes were made following the sessions, since the material of Sammy's analysis formed the basis, at that time, of a weekly case seminar, directed by Serge Lebovici at the Paris Institute of Psychoanalysis.

Following Sammy's departure for the United States, his mother, who remained in Paris with her husband, asked if she too might undertake an analysis with Joyce McDougall. This second fragment of analysis provided further insight into the genesis of psychotic disturbances like Sammy's, by revealing the intimate links that bind mother and child. Mrs Y's structure played an integral part in the disturbed nature of Sammy's object relationships and made possible retrospectively, a deeper understanding of the intense drama which Sammy re-created in the analytic situation. His life was coloured by the constant struggle to maintain his fragile identity—at the cost of suffering and solitude, and the incomprehension of those around him. We might add that he sometimes inflicted almost as much suffering on his family as he himself experienced, thus making it often impossible for those who loved him most to help him.

It seemed to us that a detailed study of the inner world which Sammy revealed in his analysis might provide a valuable contribution to the psychoanalytical understanding of child psychosis. The creation of a psychotic structure in the personality is sometimes the only way in which patients like Sammy can relate to their world and at the same time avoid the psychic dangers of catastrophic explosion, disintegration and annihilation. The study of psychotic regression, for all those who have the courage to lend themselves to such work and to identify themselves with the inner world of the psychotic sufferer, has still further value in that it provides insight into the experiences of the small infant, and, as well, enriches our knowledge of normal child development, as Klein and Winnicott have shown. Indeed, such studies give us a privileged glimpse into the universal unconscious of man, for somewhere inside each of us, Sammy's world is also our world.

It is of course inevitable that the personality of the analyst plays an important role in the material of Sammy's analysis. We must remember, however, that any research in the human sciences calls in question the personality of the research-worker. The observer who believes he is merely reporting cannot fail eventually to *interpret*, whatever technical perfection may inform his methodology.

In our initial French edition each analytic session was followed by a commentary and the book also included an extensive survey of the literature of child psychiatry and psychoanalysis relating to infantile psychosis, bringing to the attention of the French reading public the vast contributions of the Anglo-Saxon world to this subject. In the present edition the introduction is greatly shortened and no attempt has been made to survey the literature since 1960; the original references which remain have been, in many instances, revised and corrected. Commentaries have been abridged and often deleted. The clinical material has been left essentially intact.

We shall not review here, as we did in the 1960 edition, the historical evolution of the concept of infantile schizophrenia with its references to early German, Swiss and American contributions, but will confine ourselves to the statement that in France many workers have been led to abandon this concept in favour of the more general descriptive terms of 'prepsychotic' and 'psychotic childhood states'. One reason for this lies in the fact that our follow-up experience has demonstrated that many children diagnosed as schizophrenic evolve towards a pathological character-structure in adulthood rather than to chronic schizophrenic psychosis. Furthermore, differentiation between childhood schizophrenia and psychopathology related to encephalopathology of early infancy is often extremely difficult. It may be harmful to our clinical work and indeed naïve to insist on establishing clear-cut distinctions between symptoms of functional origin and those related to certain types of organic brain lesions. As Diatkine (*Revue Française de Psychanalyse*, **22**, p. 562) has shown, disturbances in object-relations particularly between mother and baby are enhanced by organic defects in the child and may thus lead to faulty maturation and developmental disharmony, and subsequently, to a psychotic structure. Our psychotherapeutic experience with such children indicates that disturbances of this kind are experienced by the child as though they were the consequence of traumatic and early frustration by the environment, even where mothering may have been adequate, in Winnicott's sense of the 'good-enough mother'. Accordingly, our psychoanalytical approach does not differ from that which we would employ towards children who present no organic disturbance.

Chapter 2 of our original book dealt with psychiatric descriptions of the various clinical aspects of psychotic states in children of different age groups. Sammy fits the group who show veritable states of motor excitation and give free verbal expression to many of their intimate fantasies. The most primitive ambivalent relations with the maternal object are sometimes expressed in open-book fashion. This is in marked contrast with the group who have apparently withdrawn interest from their environment and speak little, if at all, of their inner world.

We commented on the well-established clinical fact that certain forms of infantile psychosis are masked by pseudo-neurotic formations which present obsessional, phobic or hysterical features. In particular, the phobic-type anxieties tend to have, for the sensitive observer, a peculiar tonality, to some extent rendered 'cold', and often accompanied by precise descriptions of the phobic situations given by the children themselves, and startling in their detailed elaboration. Severe phobic anxiety in these children may sometimes become the only way of entering into contact with the world. To a certain degree, Sammy's 'Magic Face', so vividly described in the first weeks' sessions, gives us a glimpse into such phobic anxiety.

One area of developmental disharmony which we consider to be particularly worthy of study is in the field of language. Many writers besides ourselves have emphasised the vivid contrast so often displayed by these children, of a marked precocity in their vocabulary and a marked deficit in syntactical usage. This disturbance creates a tragic effect in children capable of using an appropriate vocabulary (even a highly technical, abstract or poetic one) when their sentence structure is so awkward and poor. Their self-object confusion—and fusion—is clearly revealed by their misuse of personal pronouns. These language problems inevitably distort and complicate still further the difficult object-relations of these children, creating a barrier to parental understanding in the home, as well as to therapeutic understanding in treatment sessions. The disturbance in primitive object-relations, in which we see the psychopathological basis for the organisation of childhood psychosis, can be understood from a double viewpoint: it may be the consequence of the mother's incapacity to assure from her side satisfactory early object-relations, and/or specific developmental delays and disharmonies can be the origin of frustrations in the psychological fact of the infant's experience. Furthermore, these latter frustrations may ultimately be relived by the child as though they had been consciously intended by the 'bad' maternal object.

In our 1960 edition we also discussed the interesting theoretical problems posed by the concepts of prepsychotic and psychotic states in childhood. These problems have continued to occupy the interest of certain workers in France but a discussion of the issues is beyond the scope of an English edition. All are agreed, however, that the classical descriptions of adult schizophrenia in terms of hallucination and delusion afford us little help in describing psychotic states in the ever-developing child. It is rather in the sense of an exterior reality, coloured and impregnated by the child's inner fantasy life, that we can understand more fully the psychic reality of these children. The normal evolution of a reality-sense in the infant appears to develop through his simultaneous awareness of his own body and the external world. But he becomes capable of conceptualising and recognising himself only when he can give an independent existence to others; in the beginning, to his mother. Thus 'reality' is constructed for him through a continuum of ever-widening experiences, linked with his increasing awareness of space and time. Psychoanalysis has consistently revealed the cardinal importance of the human relationship in

4

the maturation of the sense of reality—maturation which is the result of the *dialogue*, preverbal and verbal, conscious and unconscious, between mother and child, completed as the child grows older by other dialogues with subsequent love objects, in particular, the father. The latter's influence on the dialogue is, of course, present from the beginning and conveyed to the child through the medium of his mother and *her* relationship to the father.

To estimate the degree to which a given child's fantasies infiltrate and distort his sense of reality, we must attempt to communicate with him. The impossibility for the psychotic child to do this, outside of his fantasy world, is an important diagnostic sign. The psychoanalyst, with his developed capacity for identification, empathy and insight, attempts to *re-establish the dialogue*. The distortions in the child's reality-testing and perception then begin to reveal their full extent, and their meaning in the context of the analytic relationship.

Normal children differentiate between their fantasy world as elaborated in their play and the coherent verbal relation which marks daily social life. They know that their play world is an imaginary one, and they are capable of leaving it when required, to take up usual relations in the environment. In contrast, the psychotic child lives in, and loses himself in his fantasy world. He does not even understand what play is, and is incapable of the reality-oriented behaviour found in the non-psychotic child. In the young child, with his immature ego structure, fantasy normally brings about a certain alteration in his sense of reality; but a continuing 'fantasization' of reality becomes a matter of concern as the child grows older. On the one hand this translates the world into an anachronistic mirage, and on the other it leads to a progressive impoverishment of the reality-testing function of the ego. It goes without saying that in studying the troubled object-relations of the psychotic child, the defensive function of such 'fantasization' of reality shows up clearly.

In the analytic situation the transference provides an ideal setting for a detailed study of the object-relations of psychotic children. (See in this connection, the work of H. Rosenfeld, W. Bion and H. Searles). These object-relations are characterised by massive emotional impact which is subject to global variation and oscillation and coloured by a constant infiltration of fantasy, including that related to the most primitive part-objects. Fantasies of incorporating and ejecting parts of the mother's body, of sadistic attack and of disintegration are mingled with fantasies of fusion with a blissfully

5

idealised object, which in turn serves as a defence against the more frightening anxieties connected with objects (particularly the retaliatory part-object mother). Autistic withdrawal just as frequently forms part of the spectrum of defence mechanisms, in an attempt to find magical protection against destruction by persecutory objects. Such defences, typical of the psychotic ego, lead to new anxieties such as fear of a dangerous (rather than an ideal) fusion with the mother, of loss of identity, and of explosion and disintegration.

Any attempt to understand from a pathogenetic viewpoint the organisation of the psychotic ego must include reference to the earliest experiences of the infant. The psychoanalysis of young children, since the work of Melanie Klein, has greatly enriched our knowledge of the primitive fantasy world associated with these early experiences. In later studies, notably by Bion, the Kleinian group has emphasised that, in contradistinction to normal development, the elaboration of the psychotic ego is marked by excessive use of projective identification as a defence mechanism, abnormal splitting (linked with confusion of 'good' and 'bad' objects, of love and hate and of ego states), as well as destructive attacks by the ego against its perceptual apparatus, as an ultimate defence.

Sammy's analysis, although interrupted so early, is particularly rich in fantasy productions which reveal certain fundamental aspects of the genesis of a psychotic relationship. This was manifested both in the development of Sammy's transference relationship to his analyst and in the fragment of the mother's personal analysis. All through his own analysis Sammy brought forth in diverse form his anxieties of being broken or internally torn to bits and pieces. Such fantasies are typical of those which form that constellation of anxieties described by Melanie Klein as the paranoid-schizoid position. In her view, infants at moments of tension normally experience anxieties of a persecutory kind. Under their impact the primitive ego just as normally uses splitting as a temporary defence mechanism. Melanie Klein holds that optimally, in this splitting, the libidinally charged part of the self will be kept, in fantasy, in relationship with the 'good' maternal object, while the aggressively charged part of the self will be projected into the 'bad' object. These fantasies are sometimes occasioned by real experiences and at other times are linked to the psychic movement postulated by Freud as a 'hallucinated' feeding breast. To do justice to the complexity of this basic schema on the levels of external and internal objects, and subsequently to its

6

distortions in cases of psychosis, would involve detailed reference to the entire Kleinian work. Here we shall deal only with certain aspects of projective identification.

Excessive identificatory mechanisms are prominent in psychotic children and take manifold forms, but they are too unstable and too poorly integrated for the needs of normal ego and superego development. Edith Jacobson emphasises the fact that the psychotic presents difficulties which concern as much the object as himself, and in a sense this experience is analogous to that of the infant who does not yet distinguish his own body from his mother's. In her article on 'Psychotic Identification' (in *The Self and the Object World*) she writes, 'The temporary or total merging of self images finds expressions in the child's feeling that he is part of his omnipotent love objects and *vice versa.* . . .' Jacobson illustrates this description with the example of a patient whom she saw regress from normal identification to a magical identification in four stages of object-relationship—closeness, likeness, sameness, and oneness.

Projection, in the simple sense of attributing one's desires and feelings to others, has long formed part of our knowledge of psychic defence. However, Melanie Klein and her followers have studied in detail the more complicated concept of projective identification. This mechanism is vividly illustrated many times in Sammy's analysis. In this concept, split off parts of the *self* are projected onto another person—i.e. a part of the psychic structure becomes, as it were, lodged in the object. H. Rosenfeld (in *Psychotic States: A Psychoanalytical Approach*, 1964) writes:

> In the transference analysis of acute schizophrenic patients it is often possible to trace the mechanism of projective identification to its origin. I have observed that whenever the acute schizophrenic patient approaches an object in love or hate he seems to become confused with this object. This confusion seems to be due not only to fantasies of oral incorporation leading to '*introjective* identification', but at the same time to impulses and fantasies in the patient of entering inside the object with the whole or parts of his self, leading to '*projective* identification'. This situation may be regarded as the most primitive object relationship, starting from birth. In my opinion the schizophrenic has never completely outgrown the earliest phase of development to which this object relationship belongs and in the acute schizophrenic state he regresses to this early level. While projective identification is based primarily on an object relationship, it can also be used as a mechanism of defence: for example, to split off and project good and bad parts of the ego into external objects, which then become identified with the projected parts of the self.

7

(Sammy's stories of the Magic Face are an example of this, in which he reveals his desire to establish a relationship with the analyst while at the same time protecting himself against the terrors inspired by this desire.)

Thus it appears that the psychotic structure is in itself a defence against anxiety, the latter being connected with both internal and external objects. In spite of the evident and serious gaps in the defensive organisation of the psychotic ego, it seems to us that such a structure serves to protect the patient against an indescribable anxiety which is experienced literally as fatal. However, the psychotic defensive system necessarily involves interference with the autonomous functions of the ego. Conflictual investment of the cognitive sectors of the ego is usually at the origin of the developmental disharmony so often revealed in psychotic children. Thus language, in many circumstances, loses its symbolic and semantic function. Each word may be invested with the ensemble of its conflict-laden significance—often the case with Sammy. In their work on child psychosis, Diatkine and Stein (*L'Évolution psychiatrique*, 1958, p. 111) present several observations on children showing marked delay in their language development. Language capacity improved rapidly when the child could autonomise his ego after analysing, in the transference, the anxiety attached to his primitive early relationship with his mother. One young girl, encephalopathic and psychotic, had great difficulty in maintaining her own autonomy, needing constantly to control the therapist in an attempt to maintain separate identities. Her shift from mutism was followed by remarkable progress in her handling of language, and a few years later she even took up Russian as a hobby!

The earliest roots and the maturation of language are of course inevitably intertwined with the evolution of the interpersonal relationship. From the beginning there is *communication* within the primitive dyad: from the infant to the mother it is preverbal (cries, other baby sounds, facial expression, posture, etc.) and from the mother to the infant it is verbal and extraverbal (the latter including skin contact, facial expression, way of holding, rhythmic rocking, etc). It is at moments of need that the nursing infant becomes most aware of this relation and of the experiences of primitive communication which establish it. On the basis of maturational progress and of a happy equilibrium in the satisfaction of needs, he can fantasy the maternal image (probably towards the end of the first year of life) and thus

8

assure himself of the permanence of the internalised mother (as the work of Spitz has shown). In this connection it is interesting to note that Elisabeth Geleerd writes:

> The normal child is able to erect an image of his mother within his ego which enables him to be contented in her absence and which seems to be the core of his development to a mature and independent individual. The psychotic child functions only in the presence of a mother substitute (seldom his own mother) ('A contribution to the problem of psychoses in childhood' in *Psychoanalytic Study of the Child*, 1946).

The psychotic object-relationship which develops on the basis of this break in earliest communication within the mother-child unit gives a pre-eminent role to pregenital conflicts which in turn colour the specific form of the structure of the oedipal complex in the psychotic child. Lebovici and Diatkine, in their study of childhood fantasy[1] have emphasised the evolutive process to which they have given the name of 'oedipification', that is, a stage which precedes the genital oedipal complex, and in which the young child is bound to imagine that his parents' desires and relationship are the same as his own—in the first instance, desire for incorporation. The relation to the mother, inevitably ambivalent, leads the child to perceive the father purely as a protection against the dangerous mother-image. This type of oedipal structure, or 'oedipification', is a far cry from a truly oedipal organisation in which, amongst other developments, the homosexual drives attached to the father-image are integrated and form part of the secondary identification with the father. In psychotic children the oedipal structure is inevitably blocked at the early stages of 'oedipification'.

A clinical example of the latter (which at the same time demonstrates the breakdown in symbolic functioning because of the way in which language is conflictualised) is the following: Philip, nine years old, sank into a psychotic regression after the death of his father, whose leg had been amputated some months prior to his death. At the time of the first consultation Philip, now adolescent, had not spoken to his mother for several years, and had retained only isolated areas of coherent activity. In his play he chose two geographical puzzles and slowly began to talk about them. The first was constituted by the French provinces which he quickly learned to put together. While doing so he would cry out pathetically: 'France, I

[1] *Revue Française de Psychanalyse* (1954), 18.

shall reconstitute you in your entirety.' The other puzzle was composed of the nations of Europe. Philip was particularly interested in the Baltic provinces integrated into the Soviet Union (since before his illness he had read quite widely, being an intellectually gifted child). 'Poor Latvia,' he would often cry out, 'I shall deliver you from the hands of that Holy Mother Russia!' A deep psychotic anxiety in its oedipal dimension is symbolised here by Philip, and at the same time we see how adequate language functioning is impaired, because infiltrated with pregenital oedipal fantasy. A structural study of the ego of psychotic children is little advanced by descriptive terms such as 'weak ego', and demands recourse to many other approaches in order to delineate more clearly the lines of its organisation. It is important also that any study of conflictual areas must be linked with a study of the non-psychotic part of the ego. The psychodynamic considerations which we have briefly evoked here formed chapter 3 of the 1960 edition, and even in its fuller version was but an approach to this vast problem, insufficient and often unsatisfying. It is our hope that the case of Sammy, so rich in clinical detail, will stimulate the reader to view this analytic dialogue in the light of his own experience and theoretical background, and so encourage his own interest in elucidating the manifold mysteries which childhood psychosis presents to us.

In conclusion, we would like to state that we believe the analysis of psychotic children is possible and valuable. In addition it provides a significant field for research into the genesis of psychotic disorder. A recent study by Ruth Thomas ('Comments on some aspects of self and object representation in a group of psychotic children' in *Psychoanalytic Study of the Child*, 1966) confirms this point of view. If we wish to be more effective clinically we need constantly to increase our knowledge from our studies of psychoanalysis as a basic science of the human personality.

With regard to technical approaches, analysts in France have in general striven to avoid any conformist stand as to what might be *the* correct technique or theoretical approach to child analysis, and have attempted to learn from all sincere and dedicated workers in the field. In a domain where so much is preverbal, we agree with Sacha Nacht in his remarks on the psychotherapy of psychosis in the adult: 'What the analyst *is* plays a more important role than what he *says*. The authenticity of his gifts is more important than their nature.' We would simply add that research must also attempt to clarify the nature and content of interpretative work; and what we *are* depends, to a certain degree, on what we *know*. The clinical approach of the Paris Institute of Psychoanalysis has also been considerably influenced by the work of Maurice Bouvet, in particular his concept of the optimal and constantly varying 'psychological distance' that can exist between analyst and patient at any given moment, in all psychoanalyses. An ear sensitively tuned to this dimension exercises a constant influence on interpetative technique with all patients. Bouvet's clinical and theoretical work, difficult to render in a few words[1] is felt to be particularly fruitful in analytic work in the field of child psychosis, where massive projective and introjective identifications are at work coupled with intense and defused love and hate. This leads often to a flight into fusion, with a consequent loss of relational 'distance' and thus of separate identity; or, on the contrary, the same intense conflicts my precipitate the patient into a flight towards an infinite emotional 'distance', rendering communication impossible.

We hope that the reader will, in the pages which follow, be able to identify himself with Sammy and his analyst in their work together, and that he will feel a participation with each, in the poignant human drama of the analysis of a psychotic child. In this way he may then arrive at his own conclusions, make new discoveries in the wealth of clinical material, and try to formulate for himself what, and when *he* would have interpreted, in his striving to understand Sammy, and to help Sammy understand himself.

[1] It is hoped that an English translation of Bouvet's work will soon be forthcoming.

SAMMY'S BACKGROUND

SAMMY was nine and a half when he came with his parents to Paris. Dr Margaret Mahler, who had seen the little boy and his parents in New York, sent the following report:

'Sammy Y has been seen in consultation by myself and several other psychiatrists. He is a nine-year-old schizophrenic child whose intellectual functions and in particular his perceptive capacities are only moderately disturbed. His bizarre and intolerable behaviour is manifested particularly in relation to his parents, and more recently towards his small sister. He has made progress in other areas as a result of psychotherapy.'

The parents were referred in the first instance to Serge Lebovici who in turn referred them to me.

The following is taken from notes made at that time, based on two interviews with both parents and one with Mrs Y alone.

Mr and Mrs Y, rather nice-looking people in their late thirties, unusually serious in manner, seem anxious to give an exact and detailed account of Sammy. They are inclined to contradict one another from time to time when talking of Sammy's motives for his peculiar behaviour, but both make every effort to co-operate in giving a complete picture. They are not emotional in their attitude and seem to want to avoid giving any impression that they feel guilty about Sammy's illness. They are, however, anxious to let me know that Sammy is 'really ill' and that they are justified in worrying about him and being concerned over many minor aspects of his daily behaviour. They seem to head off any anticipated reassurance with regard to possible prognosis, and in fact blame various people in the past who have advised them to carry on without further intervention. For example, a psychiatrist who saw Sammy four years ago said he was mentally defective and advised the parents to prepare him to be a farm labourer.

Father, a business man who is also a creative artist, is meticulous in manner and speech. His lengthy explanations for Sammy's behaviour are sometimes difficult to follow. He gives many examples of the impossibility of teaching Sammy anything. There is an odd detachment in his presentation, perhaps because he has said it all before. He seems to have rather high expectations of Sammy from an intellectual point of view, lamenting his son's ineptitude for abstract thinking and his concentration on detail. He also complains of Sammy's failure to carry through projects once begun, such as stamp collecting. Sammy's refusal to see things as a whole is irritating to him. Nevertheless Mr Y has been exceedingly patient in his attempts to satisfy Sammy's interminable demands, and in his desire to please Sammy. He also seems to have teased Sammy quite a lot, perhaps to counterbalance all the gratifications he is obliged to furnish.

Mother has a tense closed expression. When she talks her voice is very affirmative, slightly aggressive, and she does not smile. Her eyebrows are knotted in a slight frown during the whole interview. She herself has had four years' analysis for alcoholic problems. She says she is not a maternal person, and even before Sammy was born she did not look forward eagerly to his birth. The labour was long drawn out, a breech birth, and the head was very large. No forceps. The last stage of labour lasted 14 hours. The baby was placed in incubation for several days. For this reason she did not see him at all during the first three days, but was not unduly worried. On the fourth day a nurse brought him for his first feed. He refused the nipple, and the nurse was very harsh with both baby and mother. Mrs Y felt deeply upset by her first contact with her baby and had an intense feeling of *being rejected* by him from this very moment. Breast feeding was given up and Sammy was bottle fed by nurses for the next two weeks.

Mrs Y then went to stay with her parents-in-law where Sammy was cared for by her husband's former nurse. This elderly woman took complete charge of the baby and put him on to a rigid schedule. She was a jolly person but quite lacking in sensuous qualities. Sammy's parents think it unlikely that she would ever have cuddled or rocked Sammy, but there was no doubt that she loved him and did many things to try to stimulate his interest when he was awake. He was a 'good' baby but always unresponsive to what went on around him.

The nurse left when Sammy was two months old and Mrs Y herself took over, with some supervision from her mother-in-law. Mrs Y remembers little of her impressions of Sammy during this period apart from the fact that he never seemed interested in food or people.

He only seemed to enjoy his bath. She remembers that she sometimes felt bored by him. During this time Sammy's father was in military service and returned when Sammy was three months old. He was the first to remark that the baby did not seem to respond normally to his environment. He also drew attention to the fact that when Sammy wanted to look at something he did not seem able to co-ordinate his eyes. He would turn his whole head towards the object that interested him. He did not smile at people or even appear to be aware of them. These observations surprised Mrs Y who had not been perturbed about her baby's development up till then. She had noted that he gained weight and felt that this physical progress was a sign that all was well.

All Sammy's reactions were slow and continued to be so in the months to follow. Even when he was two years old he still did not give the impression that he really looked at things. When his parents, for example, would point things out to him through the car window Sammy would turn his head and look at the pointing finger, apparently unable to throw his glance outside. He never managed to find the interesting object which was being pointed out. Even today he sees nothing that goes on around him and seems unaware of people in the street.

In reply to my questions about the early feeding situation Mrs Y says that the baby seemed to thrive on the nurse's strict schedule and it wasn't till she herself took over that she felt irritated with her baby. She could not stand the fact that he didn't enjoy his bottle and that he was very slow in drinking. On the advice of the baby-doctor she tried to get Sammy to drink out of a glass when he was seven months old. He was very resistant and she thinks that the experiment ended with the contents of the glass all getting poured down the baby's neck. She does not remember when Sammy was finally weaned, nor how he took to solids, but she thinks they were strict about it and that bottle-feeding was stopped suddenly. In general she did everything the doctor said she should do.

During the first two years Sammy would spend hours of his day in rocking back and forth and making stereotyped movements with his hands. It was always difficult to attract his attention, and she had to make extravagant gestures to get him to come to her. He never came spontaneously to anyone. Although he never put his arms round his mother's neck or tried to cuddle in any way, he liked being tickled. The only affectionate demand he ever made was that he would sometimes put his head close to an adult's hand as though seeking to be caressed.

Sammy ate alone at eighteen months, but very slowly, and often forgot he was eating. He was still being fed at the age of six by his nanny, and is today a slow and fussy eater. He goes on dawdling over his food long after others have finished. He spills a lot, never wipes his mouth, has certain ritual ways of eating and refuses many foods, for example all fruit except oranges.

Sammy regularly bathed with his mother until he was three. When she noticed that he was visibly sexually excited she discontinued bathing with him. He has always spent hours playing in the bath and it is still difficult to get him out. Even today he will play endlessly with water, and always looks guilty when he finds himself observed.

Toilet training does not seem to have been a source of particular tension. He was put on the pot at seven months, was able to control his bowels by the time he was two years old, and was completely 'clean' by the age of three. About a year later, his interest in the functioning of his sphincters seems to have been reawakened. Up till a year ago he was obsessed with the lavatory and would spend hours flushing water. Similar infantile amusements are playing with fire and burning things, with little regard for the damage this might cause.

Sammy loves showing off and takes every opportunity of showing himself naked to people who visit the family. When he was five he used often to take out his penis in front of people. Father reports that once in the Paris metro, his attention drawn by a nudge from his son, he saw that Sammy had placed his penis sticking up through a hole in a comic paper which he was holding on his knees. As Mr Y remarks, such incidents are funny when you tell them but painful to live through. Sammy also spends long hours looking at himself naked in front of mirrors. He stares particularly at his face and his behind.

Till he was six he showed no interest whatsoever in toys. His only playthings were his hands. He would talk to them for hours, gibberish talk in which he would repeat 'Dedàn Dedàn Dedàn'. Until he was seven he talked endlessly about imaginary people. He would recount long stories about these beings to friends of the family and make up songs about them at other times. Later, from seven to eight years, he would play out scenes with himself in front of the mirror and this seemed to replace the dramatic games with his hands. Not until he was eight did he ever talk of things that really existed. It was as though he lived in front of a looking-glass. Sometimes he would play out the same scenes in front of the glass. He would bow to himself saying 'How do you do, Mr Bump-Bump', etc. About this time his father took a firm hand and insisted on slowly pushing Sammy out of his imaginary world. Sammy also came to include a family of toy tigers into his life about this time. His mother would give him a new one on special occasions and the little boy became very attached to them and would talk to them for hours. But he never played with them in the ordinary way of playing. He used to place them round his bed each night and continued this habit up until last year when during a holiday in a children's camp, he discovered that other children of his age were no longer interested in stuffed toys.

According to Mr and Mrs Y, Sammy, now nine and a half, has changed very little in the last four years. In brief the things which worry them most are the following: he has never once shown either gratitude or pleasure; the moment he receives something he has wanted he no longer likes it. There is no way of punishing him; he accepts all punishments without making the slightest change in his behaviour, and indeed does all he can to provoke punishment. He makes cruel remarks to their friends; Mrs Y feels that Sammy would be delighted if they lost all their friends. He is not interested in anything, except to do everything possible to get attention. He wears his parents out with insistent questioning, and cannot be alone even for short periods (except when listening to his records). He has never been able to play with other children. With his small sister, aged ten months, he is aggressive and almost cruel. Attempts to place him in school have failed. With other children he is completely lost. He makes pathetic efforts to imitate them, but without any understanding of their games or any attempt to get into relationship with them. His only achievement is playing chess with his father. The two learned the game together and Sammy plays it reasonably well, but even here there are often many scenes. If he loses, he will sob for a long time and usually insists that the game be played and replayed until he wins. In addition, should the father ever touch Sammy's queen, the ensuing crisis is intolerable. Apart from the chess games it appears that both parents tend to put an end to those activities which Sammy enjoys. For instance, last year Sammy asked his mother to read him stories. This year she stopped doing so on the ground that he was too big and would never learn to read for himself if she continued. It was the same with bodily contacts. Since Sammy has been able to tolerate being caressed, his demands have been so great that it has been impossible to satisfy him. The parents' attitude is doubtless motivated partly by fear of the way in which he carries to excess everything he does. Although Mrs Y claims that she is rather detached from Sammy I note that she spends most of her time worrying about him.

The parents are anxious for Sammy to start treatment. They say he has had a year's psychotherapy already and loved going to his sessions. We arrange that I shall see Sammy on a five-times-a-week basis, and the parents again after three weeks. The rest is told in the session notes which follow.

THE ANALYSIS

Session (Thursday 28.10.54)

I open the door to Mrs Y and a slender frail-looking boy who stares at me fixedly behind thick-lensed glasses. Without a word or a backward look he leaves his mother behind and follows me into the consulting-room. He does not move when I invite him to sit down but stands still, his eyes roving. At my suggestion he wanders round the room looking at books and walls, then gazes vaguely out of the window before coming to perch himself carefully on the edge of his chair. I tell him there are paints, crayons and plasticine if he wants to use them, or we can just talk if he prefers. He stares at me solemnly for a moment, but as though he does not really see me.

> S. – What'll I do?
> J. M. – That's up to you.

He chooses the water colours and begins to paint with an air of serious concentration, a rather messy and indistinct picture in which brown, red and black are painted one over the other.

> S. – You want to see it? Don't you know what it is? It's a man on a horse. What would you do with it if I gave it to you?
> J. M. – Well, what do you suggest?
> S. – Oh I'm giving it to you anyway. You can do what you like with it. So come on, what are you going to do with it?

He is most insistent and I try without success to get him to tell me what he thinks would be the future of his gift. He takes another sheet of paper and begins to draw with his eyes shut. He draws in a curious fashion even when he has his eyes open, as though he were feeling round the edges of objects, reproducing what he touches rather than what he sees. In all he makes five drawings, asking me each time to guess what they are about. When I do not join the guessing game he finally tells me what they are: (1) a boat with people on it; (2) a tree falling down; (3) a volcano; (4) a horse; (5) another horse.

With eyes wide open he makes a sixth drawing which he does not explain (Fig. 1). The scene appears to be indoors. There are two armchairs on either side of a marbled fireplace, and in the same position as the chairs on which Sammy and I are sitting, which are effectively one on either side of the fireplace. But on Sammy's chair

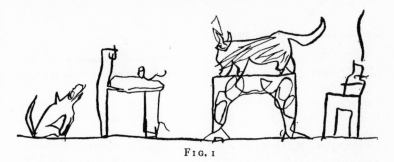

F ɪ G. 1

is sitting a small mouse, and behind it is a creature which looks like a dog. On my chair is a bottle with smoke coming out of it, says Sammy. On the mantelpiece there is a bull. (In reality there are two candlesticks with a tall candle in each.)

S.–Now please could you give me something to drink. I'm very thirsty. Oh, please. I don't want anything like orange juice. Haven't you got some milk? (He becomes most insistent.)

J. M.–Well, you can ask Hélène, the maid, to give you a glass of milk.

S.–Is it good and cold? Can it be sieved? I don't like the cream.

He drinks the milk at one gulp and then asks for more light in the room and more drawing paper. At the end of the session he is loathe to leave but finally goes off happily.

In the last drawing Sammy is perhaps showing us a first indication of his transference feelings. He is represented as a little mouse (threatened by an animal behind his chair), while the analyst is a bottle, object of oral wishes. Sammy asks for a drink just after doing this drawing. The bull on the mantelpiece, a classical symbol of virility is no doubt a reassuring one since he stands between the patient and the analyst. In other words the bull-father protects mother-bottle from the demands of Sammy-mouse, and also acts as a barrier to too close a contact developing between them if the little mouse's oral demands should be satisfied. This suggested oedipal interpretation of the role of the bull was confirmed three weeks later when Sammy broke the two candles on the mantelpiece saying that this made him feel 'much stronger'.

2nd Session (Friday 29.10.54)

Today Sammy is smiling and talking with assurance. Before coming into the consulting-room he tells his mother that she is not to wait for him in the waiting-room.

S. – 'No, no! You might hear sounds. I don't want any listening.'

He begins the session by asking many questions about other child patients I might have, how old they are, what they come for, what they do. When I tell him that I cannot give any information about others who come to see me but that I would be interested to know his ideas on the subject he finally gives up and asks if he can have yesterday's drawings.

S. – Oh, you've put the titles on. Will you always do that? Are any other children's paintings in that folder? It's all mine!

He then begins a messy water colour in which vague forms only are visible, and the colours lost by running together.

S. – Can't you guess what it is?
J. M. – You tell me.
S. – It's a boat.
J. M. – What's it doing?
S. – Sinking! And guess what those are. (He indicates a series of tall crosses on the boat.) Can't you see? They're people. They're good aren't they? I'm just as pleased with this painting as the one I did yesterday.
J. M. – And the people, what are they doing?
S. – They're going to be drowned. They're-uh-scientists.
J. M. – What are scientists?
S. – (Staring at me balefully.) They're people who try to find out things! (He leans towards me with his fist clenched.)
J. M. – (Laughing.) Like me? Am I a kind of scientist?
S. – Yes, you are!

20

He then asks that this painting be put with the others and sets about cleaning the painting box. This he does most carefully, washing it out three times. He asks various questions to determine if others would also use this paintbox, and indicates that he expects it to be kept for his exclusive use. He asks me to admire his cleaning operation.

> Today Sammy clearly wanted my exclusive attention and was curious to know who else received it. It is interesting that he projects on to his mother his own curiosity, and immediately after, tries to find out whether other children come here, and so on.
>
> His curiosity of course causes him anxiety; the inquisitive scientists who are to drown no doubt reflect what Sammy feels will happen to people who are too curious. His intensive cleaning operations at the end of the session might well represent his attempts to cope with the situation and prove that he can clean up and repair any damage done to an inqusitive analyst.

3rd Session (Saturday 30.10.54)

Sammy immediately asks to see his paintings. He then makes another painting like the first ones, with several colours laid one over the other. He says it is two men in a café. While painting he begins to talk of his father and their outings together. In particular he describes visits to a certain café where his father allows him to order whatever he wants, and he tries to find original drinks like mint sirop with lemon in it. From there he goes on to talk about Mme Cor, the nanny for Sammy and his sister.

> S.–She's so mean to me. She slaps me all the time. I don't know what to do. My parents wish she would leave, but she's still there. I do wish you'd talk to my mother about it.
> J. M.–What would you want me to say?
> S.–Well, would you care if *you* got slapped? (He clenches his fist and glares at me.)
> J. M.— Perhaps you would like to give me a slap.
> S.–And if I do what'll you do?
> J. M.–What do you imagine I'd do?

21

S. – I don't know. Well, what would you do if Mme Cor slapped you?

J. M. – I expect I'd feel angry.

S. – Oh, you're much too pretty to get angry! So what would you do if I slapped you?

J. M. – I'd tell myself that you must be angry with me.

S. – But what would you *do*?

J. M. – Well, first of all I'd ask you to tell me about it, and to tell me what it is you'd really like to do to me.

S. – I didn't say I was going to.

J. M. – No, but part of you might want to.

S. – Perhaps I might want to beat you up!

J. M. – Then perhaps you're afraid of me?

S. – Yes, you might kill me!

J. M. – You don't trust me.

S. – Oh no! I don't at all.

Sammy then returns to the subject of Mme Cor and her ill-treatment of him and begs again that I speak to his mother about this. 'Please do something. No kidding, it's very serious!'

It is the end of the session and I accompany Sammy back to the waiting-room. I tell his mother as requested that Sammy wishes me to talk about the ill-treatment he feels he is suffering at the hands of Mme Cor. She turns an astonished gaze on Sammy and exclaims, 'But Sammy, how could you! Why, she is just wonderful to you. In fact she spoils you.'

Sammy turns to me grinning and dances up and down, shouting, 'Ha, ha, fooled you! You believed it didn't ya?!!'

> This joke gave Sammy the chance to turn the tables in the analytic situation, and is no doubt one way of controlling his fear of, and defence against, his transference desires. It is also interesting that Sammy could not give his true feelings about Mme Cor to whom he is obviously very attached. His mother had to express his feelings for him.

4th Session (Monday 1.2.54)

Sammy begins by looking into my eyes and singing, 'The face, the face, the pretty little face.' He starts to paint but keeps up his invented song with infinite variations on the same theme. He starts spontaneously to talk about his painting.

> S. – This is a magic face. See it changes colour! (He is at this moment passing a wash of water colour for the third time.) This face has no body, just long feelers, one longer than the other. It's half a man and half a lady. It walks down the streets and it can do anything it likes. It could do everything before it was born. A face, a pace; a face a pace; a funny little face ... etc.

Sammy is much more excitable today, and spends the whole session talking in a rather dissociated way. At times he speaks dramatically as though he were making announcements or reading aloud from a story. I am unable to remember his flood of words but the recurrent images make reference to hands with fingers chopped off, people with no feet, no bodies and so on.

When he lays down the paint brush towards the end of the session (the painting now unrecognisable under its many coats of colour) he shouts: 'Put that down before something kills you!'

He then begins splashing water on the carpet and imperiously demands more water. When I make no comment he pours the remaining paint water into various objects in the room, and looks at me as though trying to study my reactions. I have the feeling that for the first time he has somewhat relaxed his control of himself in front of me, particularly in regard to his attempts to communicate. Many of his thoughts and even the words he uses are disordered and he no longer seems concerned that I should understand. At the end of the session he catches up his earlier more careful behaviour. When he rejoins his mother he says in a loud stage whisper, 'Tell her my pet name for her.' His mother looks rather embarrassed and says, 'He calls you Dougie.' Going down the stairs he turns and calls out, 'Dougie, I think you're very beautiful.'

In the excited atmosphere of this session Sammy talks fluently and rapidly, albeit in a rather chaotic way. He passes without pause from the analyst's face to the frightening Magic Face with it's bisexual constitution and it's long feelers. He gives the impression of being under the sway of a terrifying fantasy whose intensity disturbs his capacity to communicate. The Magic Face expresses not only castration anxiety but also a fear of disintegration. In addition we notice that the chopped-up Magic Face can retaliate and chop up others, including the analyst who might get killed if she touches it.

It is of interest that Sammy is able to regain his control towards the end of the session, showing the strength of his defence against the unconscious fantasies struggling for expression.

Protected by his mother's presence and implicit permission, Sammy can reveal that he has a pet name for me, and that he finds me 'very beautiful'. (This as we saw in the last session means that I will not get angry.)

5th Session (Tuesday 2.11.54)

S. – Today I want to write a story about the Magic Face. Can I tell it to you and you take it down? You see I can't write much in English. I only know a little bit of French.

Sammy does, however, write the title of his story on the page on which he orders me to take his dictation, and accompanies it every so often with vague pencil drawings representing human faces or animals. Once or twice he attempts to write a few words himself, but soon gives up. On each new page he draws an irregular outline within which I am to write his story. All attempts to get him to talk are in vain. He insists on my writing down every word and dictates the following:

'This face is very magic, and that is why it is called the Magic Face. This face can do anything it wants to. If you ever saw it you would be surprised because it can do so many things. For instance it can kill anybody it likes, and make dead people come to life. It could think and talk and everything it wanted before it was born. And this Magic Face can change itself into lions and tigers and hippo-popotamus and ants [sic] and uncles. This face is half of everything, half hippo and half tiger, half kangaroo without a second leg, half elephant without a trunk and just like a dog that didn't have no tail and no front paw. So this face is a mongrel to a person just like a dog is a mongrel to other dogs.

'Magic Face can be very frightful sometimes, but once in a while, every Christmas, it makes a smile once in a while, but not all the time. And this face is the magicist face in the world. This face is a big face not a small face. No one ever saw it in the world before. If ever it comes people will be most surprised. Even though it won't really come people can dream about it and think about it as a fairy tale.

'This face is fifty-one years old and it is twenty-one feet high and nine feet round, and this face never dies. This face lives in a place with many people around. And all these people you can see in dreams and believe in tales like the Magic Face which lives in a place with nobody around except thirty people.

'The place is a face but nobody knows why, but I shall sigh if I know why. HI! said the Face to a tiny little man who only had one hand. But the Face feels sorry for him because he has no chin. Now this man saw a baboon as he was looking at the moon. But now the moon shines low down. As the trees look brown because it's autumn now. How shall I find my way home if the Face doesn't find me?

'And far far in the distance he saw the Magic Face running as she could—because it's half lady and half man. So if ever she had enemies she could turn her face into a broken radio so then the enemy wouldn't bother her. When the enemy saw the broken radio they would pay no attention and just keep on with their war.

'And little Chipsie-Hopsie the rancoon after he jumped down off the moon well, Mrs Magic Face saw her and said, "What is this? What is this? Jumping over the moon! I just can't stand it. This scares me out. I shall chase him out of the way, all the way back into his tree. And now I'm going to turn into a tiger." '

On this page Sammy then made a rapid sketch. In one corner there is a half-moon and beside it the sun. Underneath a sort of dog and a primitive human figure with something resembling a tree alongside.

Page 4. Title, 'How I Turn Myself Into a Tiger.'
'I changed one of my hands into a paw, so then I look like a face with one hand and one paw. Then I put up one of the skins I have on my face and it looks exactly like a tiger ear. And with my tail I change into a tiger's tail—really like one. And then my other two paws jump out. The things that jump out is part of my intestines. And then I look and see that one paw is missing.

'Now she looks at herself. "I'm a real tiger now." She chased the racoon into a tree singing Dee de dee de dee (here Sammy sings and requests that I kindly take down the tune in musical notation!).

25

'Now the tiger who is Miss Bradburg, the Face's name, chases the little thing into its tree, and that was the end of this, the end of it for this story. And this face went all the way home and changed itself into a bird into its second storey window. The house had 4932 storeys.'

The drawing on this page clearly represents a very large animal springing upon a very small animal. The movement is dynamic and the drawing more detailed than the others.

The text continues on page five as follows:

'So this house is 17 storeys high. The face, the pace, is the face for me. (Sammy asks me again to note the music.) The Face cuddled into bed on this long day. As she never got tired she stayed awake all night and looked at books. So the Face stayed in the house for ever. It was the end of her adventurous life. She'd had enough. She decided to turn herself into a regular person, and would live till 80 or 90 like everyone else. She never had an enemy and all the people in the village were her friends. An old lady of 51 with real hands and real legs. Never again a magic face. She turned all the magic into regular things because now she wanted to be a regular person. She walked in the street, a regular lady with a cane, because all the magic she had, had excited her too much. And all her friends came to her house. She had a great big party, so much fun, never displeased. She lived on long and happily, never got sick and died at a regular age. A happy lady in a town, and a good lady.'

On this last page Sammy has drawn a house with a very pointed roof and standing on the chimney there is a little figure wearing a sort of helmet.

Towards the end of this session he asks permission to take his story home, saying he wants to show it to his parents. He is so insistent that I finally allow him to take it on condition that he bring it back next day, which he accepts. He makes a great fuss about leaving and I tell him that he finds it difficult to separate and perhaps in his desire to take the story home is trying to take something which is part of him and me away with him.

Sammy dictates his story in a state of barely controlled excitement, and talks with surprising rapidity. At times he is using words as objects rather than as a means of communication. (Some weeks later, he himself draws attention to his difficulty in communicating with others if they do not understand the personal meaning he gives to certain words (Session 40).) Here he is making an immense effort to cope with and control the anxieties underlying the main themes by moulding them into a reasonably coherent story, a creative attempt which is more successful than his earlier expression through painting.

The themes gradually unfold, beginning with the Magic Face as an omnipotent person, a dangerous killer, who in turn becomes mutilated, then a body broken into pieces. This destroyed object becomes itself a destroyer. As Sammy's anxiety mounts, the details he gives of the Magic Face's relation to its objects are reminiscent of the fantasies of frightening part-object relationships, of a fusion between a destroyed and a destroying object.

Sammy struggles to deny and control the upsurge of his frightening fantasies by insisting that what he is describing is only a fairy-tale. He also tries to keep the terrifying Face and all it symbolises within bounds by giving it definite dimensions. Introducing into the story 'the little man' who is lost and has no chin, he speaks in the first person, which suggests that he himself is appealing for help. At this point, it is of interest that the Face becomes a woman, a frightening and damaged figure (as all maternal figures seem to be for Sammy). The castrated mother-figure becomes less terrifying when she is turned into someone who is 'half man and half woman'. Here, the drama projected onto the face clearly conceals archaic primal scene imagery.

In the next phase, when face-to-face with the little animal (the little man, Sammy), 'she' turns into a tiger. It is at this moment of utter confusion over identities and primal scene magic that the Magic Face becomes frightened and renounces it's omnipotence, 'because all the magic had excited her too much'. She returns to normality and becomes a whole 'regular' person. [Sammy no doubt needs her this way so that he himself can become a whole and 'regular' person whose troubling magic, his magic defences, will not frighten him.] Throughout all these themes, Sammy not only reveals his fear of losing his identity but also the extent to which he must struggle against the projective character of the fragmented objects. When these objects themselves become invested with destructive power, the Magic Face represents the fusion of Sammy and his analyst. By this magical means he attempts to escape the destructive relationship which is felt to be so dangerous for both.

The fairy-story is a reassuring one since it allows Sammy to externalise frightening fantasies which were already arousing a good deal of anxiety in the previous sessions. Furthermore, it is undoubtedly reassuring for him to find that the analyst can survive these attacks. She can be used as an object against which the most primitive fantasies can be acted out.

This session not only shows the chaos Sammy feels as a result of his confusion about his identity, but also reveals anxiety arising from his terror of disintegration, and gives some insight into the methods by which he attempts to escape these anxieties. The fact that he spent the entire session *dictating* was also an attempt at keeping his anxiety within bounds; and from now on, every session for some months to come was spent in Sammy's dictating to me, while each new session began with a demand that I read the old one back to him.

6th Session (Thursday 4.11.54)

S. – Another story today.

J. M. – I was very interested in yesterday's story. And I've been wondering who the Magic Face is.

S. – Shut up!

J. M. – I wonder if you're a bit scared to talk about this story, Sammy?

S. – Well now, if you want a conversation—I'm just not going to join in, see?

He orders me to start writing immediately. 'This story is called "The Blizzard".' He again draws a line down the middle of the page in which I am to write the text, while he will add a drawing on the other side.

First page, ' "Well", said Mr Mannering, "I'm not going to stand living in my old house. I'll go and build in the woods and be with other animals and make friends with them. Just as well see birds, monkeys, and kangaroos which I like very much, said the little plump man. I'll find a wood and start a small house." And so he did. "That's a fairly good house," he said. "Not the best I could make, but not the worst. My little house has a fireplace, a chimney, a window and a man which is me. So in my house there's just one of each, not two of the same thing. Well, so my day goes a little happier. I'll go down to the farm to be with the horses and cows and talk to the farmer, who is an old man of 49." So he walked off into the deep woods on the way to the farm. And he liked it a lot in the woods with the little animals, chipmunks, cows and canary birds.' (The drawing accompanying this page shows a man who seems to be running, and behind him is a roughly sketched-in house.)

Page 2. 'Of course they don't have tigers and lions because I know these woods very well. As he got out in the open he found himself right by the farm. And the farmer waved at him, without an answer. There was Miss Jerry Hamsten who had three children and a father and Miss Scraps the Patchwork Girl. And Princess Ozma was not far. She was head of the town and she had these children—Princess Dorothy, and Ojo who happened to be the man on the farm. Ojo felt so sorry when he found out that his Uncle Unc got the life powder, and so his body turned into marble. Ojo felt real sorry for him. "How am I going to find Unc? I can't do a thing for him."' (This text is adorned with another house drawing, and two figures which appear to be male and female.)

Page 3. 'In the story of the lost Princess of Oz, he happens to be not in it. But he's in the Patchwork Girl. The magician turned the room upside down, and Ozma was imprisoned. A little boy finds her in a peach pip. And afterwards, flip-flop, they all walked home. That's the end of that part of the story. Now this second part, Unc got turned into marble-brick with the powder of life. The phonograph came to life too. They all hated this phonograph. And the Woosie was there, all in the wood. A wooden horse who could shoot fire out of his eyes. Say a magic word if you want me to shoot fire! Waskiboochiwoochy. Way up in the trees a voice said ooooooo. Whooooooo they heard again. And again they said the magic word.' (Sammy's drawing represents the wooden horse shooting flame from his eyes. He looks very wooden and square.)

Page 4. 'So the Woosie shot fire out of his eyes, and the fence fell flat on its side. Woosie escaped. He had wooden feet and three hairs on the end of his tail. They all pulled his tail but didn't succeed in getting one hair out. They needed it to make Ojo's Unc come to life.

Striked lightening made something cry inside. Once they saw three men sitting around the fire. And no one knew what it was. A face a pace a pretty little face came in the sky. Everyone was surprised, and didn't know who she was. It was the Magic Face. And they saw it. The same lady with the cane, and they all said she'd had enough. The face the pace the dirty little face. There was once a big blob of clay on the ground. Miss Scraps kissed it. It was Princess Ozma. And Ojo found his Unc who stopped being marble-brick, and hugged him. The face the pretty little face. No one knows but the face is there not here. It's behind the tree. I am the wolf and I am the lion. And now I shall get you, said a voice from the distance. The chipmunk got so scared. He ran from the tiger and the lion who were licking each other's tongues. The fox's guts were going to be bitten out by somebody.' (The few sketch lines which follow the text are vague and resemble the Magic Face.)

    S. – You got a pretty face.
J. M. – Perhaps I am the Magic Face?
    S. – Do you know who it is?
J. M. – No. But I thought it might be me. You aren't too sure what you think of her, whether she's good or bad.
    S. – You're pretty like a film star. Why are you so pretty? Do you think you're pretty?

It is the end of the session and Sammy objects vociferously to leaving.

    S. – No, no! Don't go!! There's something very important to tell you.
J. M. – You can tell it tomorrow.
    S. – No. Now! It's about school. I'm going to a school class.

While talking, Sammy throws his arms about me and seems about to kiss me, then changes his mind, starts to tear at my clothes, and looks rather as though he wanted to bite me.

J. M. – Sammy, I don't think you're at all sure what you feel like doing towards me at the moment. And perhaps you are trying to see what I shall do. But you do have to go now.

(He grabs me round the legs with his arms, and we get ourselves somehow or other into the waiting-room. Just at the door Sammy straightens up and begins to act in a more normal fashion. He runs back into the consulting-room once more and shouts, 'The face the pace the pretty little face.')

Today, in his flight from anxiety aroused by the transference Sammy takes refuge once more in fantasy, and keeps control of the analytic situation by continuing to dictate. As the stories unfold life itself gets dangerous; human beings are transformed into inanimate objects, and conversely, using fantasied magic power, the child brings inanimate objects to life. The 'powder of life' makes the gramophone into a living thing, while the uncle is turned into marble. Bad or terrifying aspects of the Face turn up in the Woosie's 'eyes which can shoot fire'.

Frightened by his omnipotence, Sammy protects himself by stressing the good aspects of the Magic Face and projecting them onto the analyst, the 'regular lady', of the previous session. He now feels safe enough to approach the most terrifying fantasy which is an evocation of the primal scene: the lion and tiger lick each other's tongues while the fox's guts are torn out.

When the analyst suggests that she herself is the Magic Face in both its reassuring and its frightening aspects, Sammy reacts strongly, showing excited erotic feelings tinged with ambivalence. This is understandable since Sammy has projected onto the Analyst-Magic Face many of his 'bad' feelings as well as good images of himself. In the next session he asks to have his story read back, no doubt seeking reassurance that he can recuperate all that has been projected.

7th Session (Friday 3.11.54)

S. – Read me the story of the Magic Face.

I try to get Sammy to talk about it but my efforts are met with 'Enough of that now! Go on! Oh, you are terrible; I'm not here to answer questions.'

The story read, Sammy demands a glass of milk, and on this occasion pushes the bell himself to call Hélène into the room. She brings it, and Sammy says cheekily, 'Merci ma vieille.' ('Thanks old thing!')

S. –Now read the second story.

Again he avoids any discussion of the story but instead questions me insistently about my other patients, whom he supposes to be all children.

S. –Oh, you won't even answer a question, You're that mean! Well I guess I'll write another story. Write it down. It's called 'The Earth and Its Animals.'

I am the brother cow said a voice. And I am the little calf in the family. I'm the fox, brother fox. And a voice far far away said I'm the dragon. And I'm the son of dragon. But I am the FATHER said a very loud voice. And I'm going to make this ground shake. I'm the big thing which shakes the ground. I'm called Droblia Terrias and I shall knock down thirty trees. And that scared the rat and the rabbit and the chipmunk and the great big polar bear and the racoon. And even the MAGIC FACE, who was running around the thirty trees. The Magic Face was jumping over the animals—the vomiting hippopotamus and pregnant rhinoceros and the elephant who had four paws and awful diarrhoea. And the Magic Face flew across the forest and stamped on a canary bird and broke its beak off. The vomiting hippos and the pregnant rhino and the lions and tigers with big fluffy behinds all ran away. Not one was left. The bird with the beak was killed by the Magic Face. And after, they all gave their great big rumpus. The Magic Face was yelling holy harrious. All the animals roared and galloped and shook the thirty trees. The chipmunk jumped on the vomiting hippopotamus's back. Then the hippo jumped over the elephant's back. The elephant gave a big roar, wah! and then the great big dragon with the biggest tail was so angry. Thunder came from the sky and lightening and erupting volcanos. So all the animals pounced on the dragon until his guts flew out, and his heart. So he flew flat on his face, dead.'

S. –(To me) Now don't you stop writing.

The vomiting stopped. The diarrhoea and all the other animals with troubles stopped. And a lady's eyeballs popped out from the sky. And lightening all fell down to pieces. The biggest rumpus the animals ever heard. Rocks were breaking. They killed the poor elephant. Soon the oceans of all the world swept over all the land. And the earth was covered with water. Ice fell from the sky, the sun came out and the water began to boil. All the animals were in dreadful pain. The sun was coming closer. There was fire. Soon all was death. Just the earth spinning alone. Everything was death. Just the ground burning and the water boiling. The earth was getting smaller and smaller till Crash! Bang! Crash! The earth hit the sun. And it burst with a tremendous explosion. There was not a living thing. What was left of the earth all came from the sun. Nothing but ashes. So that was the end of the earth.

And now the sun was only with the eight planets instead of nine. What happened to the earth was very sad. Just a little music came. Even the Magic Face was dead. It was the only thing that could kill her. Then they could see the face in the sky. It was the Virgin, and her face said 'Since the earth blew up there'll never be another earth ever again.' And that was the end of the adventurous planet. The sky got bluer and bluer and the Face went away. Then the sky was very peaceful without the earth. No living thing in the universe. Not on this planet earth. And there was silence except for the clouds. Then thunder and lightening came. But never it came as hard as it did on this earth. So the sky was peaceful.

Far, far away they saw clouds. A tremendous storm which swept across the universe, then the sun came out. It was too bad there was no more earth. Without an earth the sun shined all the time on the other planets. The rest of the universe was just silent. So in the earth's places just gasses, a little mist and smoke. After that nothing. Just an empty space.

Sammy indicates that this is the end of the story. I open my mouth to speak, but he cuts me off short.

> S. – Well now, if you want to make a conversation out of this then I'm going!
> J. M. – Afraid of having conversations with me?
> S. – Enough! Now here's another story. Go on. Write!

And a soft wind blew by. It was a nice wind. And the sun shone. The night came. The stars shone. Night and the soft wind came again. Except for the earth and the animals that got killed, this world was a good world for all the people who lived in it.

In reply to my questions Sammy said, 'You want to know too much! But what would you do if the earth exploded really?' He refuses to divulge what he thinks either he or I would do in such a situation. At the end of the session he leaves unwillingly.

> I note that he is getting a little more dictatorial each day; while recounting his cosmic fantasies he is in a state of intense excitement but the anxiety which accompanies them makes him take refuge in dictating rather than talking. He also keeps a distance between us by asking Hélène to bring the milk directly. Nevertheless the glass of milk arouses his curiosity and jealousy of his analytic siblings. It is also highly probable that the drinking of the milk gives rise to the images of the vomiting hippo, the elephant with diarrhoea and (what is undoubtedly an unconscious equivalent for Sammy) ideas of pregnancy. Anxiety about primal fantasies emerges more and more clearly as the session proceeds. In order to escape from these, including the frightening Analyst-Magic Face, Sammy turns to a powerful father-figure for protection, (projected onto the 'voice'). It is then that his identification with the mother-figure in the pregenital images of the primal scene leads to a fantasy of cosmic chaos. The fact that the stories are kept and read back when he asks for this, reassures him nevertheless. It is tempting to suppose that the 'adventurous planet' which came to a tragic end is Sammy himself who, to a large extent, has given up his relationship with the external world.

8th Session (Saturday 6.11.54)

Sammy immediately begins to dictate a story, carefully avoiding any direct conversation. He is as frightened as he is fascinated by his fantasies; he breaks off his dictation and asks me first of all to re-read the story of the Magic Face. When I discuss his anxiety his answer is ready.

> S. – Well now if we're going to talk, I'm off. Enough! Another story. Please write! This story is called 'Captain Jeroff'.

On the first day of June they had these pirates who were going to sail on a big adventurous sailboat. And before they started their sailboat they stayed in dock for four days. Anchors picked up

34

ropes hauled up and the captain steering the boat. There was a man named Ludwig on the boat and he said he was a composer who wanted to write some music for them. He said I shall write my Fifth Symphony now. And now I'm writing it, (To me) Will you please write a few notes of music on a stave with treble clef. (He examines this carefully and adds a few 'notes' of his own.) And Mrs Ludwig Beethoven saw her husband's head being knocked down. The ship started sinking. Trees falling. Ceiling falling down on the ship. The piano broke down in the Fifth Symphony and the melody book got torn up by a bad pirate. The pirate hit Mrs Beethoven on the head with his gun. Water sploshing and the world blew up. It didn't really. It was just a daydream somebody dreamed.

All of a sudden they saw a little horse kicked from the sea. Fire was streaking from the sky. Fire, fire, fire! Get me here! I'm a bad man! Now thirty people were on top of the ship which was half broken. Now the world was shaking and the ship turned on its backside. The vomiting hippopotamus, and the broken radio that was sitting on a stump, fell into the water. And even the Magic Face turned in circles. The sky was red green blue and purple. Two paint brushes crossed each other in the sky. Queenie the Evil Horse, jumped from the sky and made a big splash. They saw her feet kicking out of the water. A big rock banged her on the head and killed her. Thirty knives fell into the ocean and went through the earth. Fire, fire, fire said a voice in the sky. Explosion of atomic bombs. What saw them? Nothing! Even though nothing does not hit nothing. Land broke! The world was spinning on its axis. You, said a voice in the sky, don't get in my way or I'll kick you out on board— if there is any board. No! No! Don't whip me on the behind. I'm *not* the vomiting hippopotamus! I'm *not* a hypochondriac. I don't worry about hospitals and things! Just get on with your business and no questions! (This was said to me as though I had spoken to him.)

S.–Now don't start any sort of conversation! (I remain silent.) Well did you *like* that story? (I open my mouth to speak and he roars me down.) Dee dee dee da da da! Now just write that will you?

And I'm going to kill you said a small voice far away. I'm a small chipmunk swimming over thirty hippopotamuses in the sea. Somebody's eyeglasses, liver, guts and kidneys popped out of the sky at one time. The laughing hippopotamus didn't care for it much coming out of its tail. And no one knew why I should sigh. But you know why. And I should die if you should say why, said a voice in the sky. A fish, a baboon and a lovely racoon.

The Magic Face said to the lady, would you like to take my place. (To me: The Magic Face was nice about that wasn't she?) What shall I do? I get so bored said the little boy to his grandmother. But why do I sigh? The sun shone on all the people in the boat and the hippo laughing. They all went in their dens for a nice cuddle-night, a warm night's sleep. Now the music comes up for you for me. But why shall I say something for you? 'No, don't cry,' said a voice.

No one knows why everyone went home. How is it? The land got very boring for all the people in this world, and so happy, never knew they had such a good adventure. All so happy and so glad, once more.

> Following the primal scene anxieties of last session we seem this time to have confused and technicoloured images of pregnancy. Sammy's little sister was born only last year and we can detect in the images of 'the vomiting hippopotamus', 'the little horse kicked from the sea (Queenie the Evil One who gets killed), and the 'liver, guts and kidneys' which popped out, some idea of Sammy's fury and his anguished imagining during this event. That Sammy does not want the analyst to talk about such things is understandable. When I open my mouth to speak he tells me to shut up as though afraid I am going to give him back all the troubling feelings and ideas he is trying to get rid of. He does not even wish to carry such terrifying images away with him. Before leaving he restores the situation so that everything is 'all so happy and so glad once more'.

9th Session (Monday 8.11.54)

Sammy gets to work right away on a new story as though there were not a minute to lose.

S. – This story is called 'Ubink'.

> Once there was a little rat who tried to jump from one tree to another but didn't quite make it and he saw a little rabbit who was

trying to get into his hole but didn't care for the chipmunk tail in the way.

'Ha ha ha,' said an old man. I'm not going to stand for this all of the time, even though there's so much bushes in my way. Now I heard something in the skies said a young man who was walking right besides him. The old man didn't even notice it. They saw thirty tents far far away and they knew the Jerry Chipsiehops who lived in it. And there was an ocean not far from these tents. And there was a great big jungle not far from the ocean and the tents. Inside, they had funny people who had thirty noses and forty hands and three thousand and nine hundred and forty-two feet. And one time as the old man was walking in the woods he saw a little thing and tried to kiss it. And the little thing said, 'Ha ha, don't try to kiss me'. The old man saw it was a great big boar and he ran away from it. It started chasing him on all four legs, chasing the man back to his home. He would never never kiss anything like that again. He wasn't thinking that the jungle had wild animals. So he ran so fast that he tripped over a tube-stone and fell into an inkwell with thirty miles downward of water. It was really beating him up. The man realised he had a knife in his pocket. So he took it out and killed the boar between the two guts. 'Now I've killed a real boar and I am proud of myself. I shall just tell my great old mother I killed a boar.' Before he got out of the ink he thought he might try to clean himself. He pulled the boar out and threw him by some rocks so people wouldn't have to see it in front of them. So he cleaned himself in the ocean, a nice swim with his clothes on, then hanged them on the branch of a tree. He walked to his house nakedly, put nice clean clothes on while the others were drying off. He felt quite good at not being all wet. So he walked to his mother's house and told how he killed the boar. And his mother gave a big sigh of worry. And he told that he kissed this thing and that the boar chased him and he tripped over the tube-stone and fell in the inkwell and how he killed the boar with a knife which he found in his pocket. 'You are a good man. I'm proud of you. I'll buy you new clothes. You changed just for me. I thank you quite a bit,' said his mother. They found a blue shirt, grey pants, brown belt and shoes. He was proud and said, 'Now I'm a real man, just like I was at thirty, even though I'm about forty.' And he felt quite good to kill the boar. Quite a bit of muscle to kill it. He just had a little bitten finger but not much damage. Just a little pain in his bones.

37

He realised he would never penetrate that forest. On the right, there was the jungle. On the left was the nicest forest place for walking. After, he went back to his beautiful home, hugged and kissed his mother and turned round in circles.

Perhaps the week-end break helped to stimulate the oedipal jealousy themes of this session. In any case some light is thrown on the way in which Sammy draws closer to his father in an attempt to cope with anxieties about the mother-relationship. But the anxiety about his homosexual wishes is equally intolerable. In the story the return to the mother is acutely anxiety-making also, since she represents the danger-ous jungle into which he must not penetrate, because she hides inside her not only the old man (father) but wild animals (Sammy's own dangerous oral and anal impulses and perhaps other babies). Dangerous contact fantasies are re-vealed in the 'little thing' which when kissed turns into a horrible boar. Although he 'goes back to his beautiful home, hugs and kisses his mother and turns in circles' Sammy does not readily tolerate this wonderful contact.

10th Session (Tuesday 9.11.54)

S. – Quick, more stories.

J. M. – You know, Sammy, I think you like to tell stories partly so we won't talk about what they mean.

S. – Well, uh, well (shoots an astonished glance at me as though he suddenly understood my remark). Well you just write anyway! This is the story of Uk. Chapter one! Uk was a man and Miss Uk was a lady. Uk Suddy was a little girl and Uk Bloody was a little boy. Chapter two: Once a long long time ago there were three children and they were all six years old and they had no home to go to. Chapter three! Once there were three animals in a cage. No one took care of them and they all died . . . . . .

The 'chapters' go on in this depressive vein up to chapter fifteen where Sammy is visibly drawing on the details of my consulting-room for his inspiration, e.g. 'there was an old fireplace and that fell down, then there were some lamps and a couch and a chair beside it which all fell down and the old lady heard them and couldn't do a thing about it'.

J. M.–Sammy I think you are telling me that you have many troubled thoughts in which everything is sad or breaking up and you are afraid I can't do a thing to help *you*.

After this remark Sammy began to shout out numbers and then recounts ten more 'chapters' all containing pictures of rejection and depression. The last one is 'No one knows why says a voice in the sky. And if I knew why then I would die.' Sammy gives me the impression that on one hand he longs to know more but that knowledge is equated with death. The flight from death takes the form in the transference of a flight from anything that I might tell him. It is possible that what must not be 'known' is the sexual mystery of the primal scene and the truth about the birth of his little sister; it is all linked with the question of curiosity, which as we have already seen in the very first sessions, leads to death.

11th Session (Thursday 11.11.54)

S.–Next story. Let's get cracking! This story is called Knockerlopp. Hey what's the matter with you?

He kicks the table violently. I have the feeling that my remarks about his urgent need to tell stories when we talked of it at the last session might have given him the impression that I rejected his stories, and perhaps too that I was attacking his defensive relationship with me via the stories. I told him that I found the stories interesting, and that no doubt it was important for him to feel that he could always think up lots of new ideas for stories.

S.–Did you like them *really*?
J. M.–You didn't think I would?
S.–Oh well—let's get on with this one. Can you write French? Good. Now this story is Knockerlopp.

'It was you' said a voice. She was so funny. Her French was funny. She lived in the South of France where everyone spoke French. (From here on Sammy dictates in French of which the following is a literal translation.) Come here everybody. I want you to make your houses very clean. And make your beds please. And you, don't you annoy people, the lady said to a little boy who annoyed everybody. After that the old man wanted to visit her. 'Bonjour Madame' says he in the best French he knew and with an English accent. She replied, 'Bonjour Monsieur, I see you have long hair, and I know that your wife is about to have a baby hippopotamus.' The man was very angry with her and slapped her then ran home. (Sammy switches to English and indicates that the story concerns him and me.) The young man said to his mother that he didn't have a good conversation with the lady. She was quite pretty but not as nice as he had expected, and his mother who only knew one word in German said 'Danke' to him. And the mother and the plump hairy young man walked down to the lady's place to find out why she was so bad. 'If you want the lady to be nice', he said to his mother, 'just you be nice to her.' The lady was so angry she said, 'Would you just try to get out of here. Sortez de ma maison!' So the man and his mother moved to Paris. So this man and lady saw a lady whose name happened to be Mme Blank. (Sammy begins to describe my appearance.) She had white earrings and brown hair and had a blue suit with fur on it and a wrist watch and a lamp that didn't work so well, and clay and water colours. Mr Blank used these with her. She thought her fur collar was so nice. Mr Blank who is sitting in a red chair thought it is nice in this room. There was an old maid who worked for them and her name was Hélène. These people were English and the maid was French. Mr Blank was nine, and the lady was twenty or twenty plus perhaps. And in that room they had red flowers and a white fireplace. The lady was writing a story and the little boy was dictating it. She had a blue and silver pen that sometimes got out of ink. White earrings, finger nails polished and her initials were J. M. The boy was S Y. So they were very glad to get away from that lady who spoke French. Once she went to Mme McD. and said (the story continues in French), 'Go! Get out of this apartment or I'll give you a slap!'

The two got scared and went head over heels out in the street. She whipped them and got so crazy she didn't know what language she was speaking. Well said a voice in the sky, the earth's going to fall, the chair and the lamps will break. And no one knows why. The face, the pace, the pretty little face. Good morning Madame, don't cry for me. And the lady came home with a big walking-stick. Ha ha said a big voice in the sky. Ho ho said a small voice. But I shall kill you for a million dollars if you will give me the money. And that was the end of them! (Here Sammy switches back to English and asks me to read out his story which I do.)

S. – Your French is horrible, worse than my mother's, and she has a terrible accent! You know, Dougie, something good is to happen tonight. I'm having dinner with Mme Cor. (This was regarded by Sammy as a very great privilege, since normally he ate dinner with the family.)

The fact that I had told Sammy last session that I found his stories interesting while it made him pleased probably also frightened him. This time he creates a certain distance between us first by talking in French and second by introducing into the story his mother who thanks him when he says he doesn't like the lady; i.e. the analyst.

He turns to a paternal image as protection against the oedipal material (the woman pregnant with a hippopotamus) and also against the angry female image itself. The bad images intermingle with the pleasant ones of the mother-analyst figure. When 'Sammy Blank' is getting on too well with 'Dougie Blank' the fierce female image drives them both down the stairs. Sammy's ego is not strong enough to tolerate intense positive feelings without recourse once more to this terrifying imago. Various psychotic defences now come into play but they seem inadequate to combat the terrors of disintegration and 'the voice from the sky' which once again brings death.

12th Session (Friday 12.11.54)

S. – Hey, you're wearing the same clothes you had on the first time I came. Dinner was no good last night. Mme Cor was nervous on account of her sister who just died.
J. M. – Mme Cor talked to you about it?
S. – Will you just take down another story right away, and shut up! 'City Stories.'

When I got to New York from Paris it seemed strange with all the buildings so high, and I'm not used to it after being in Paris. But when I got there I felt quite happy, because I knew it was my country and no one spoke French. And I came to New York from a camp I

41

was at and I didn't like it. My apartment was big like a studio, eleventh floor, fifteen stories, and I went to a nice school there where I had friends. Five of them. And it was quite nice with children to play with, and around this place I don't have any. So I like New York better than Paris. And the traffic is more there and a big river called the Hudson. And when I came back from this awful camp I had so much friends. The next camp I liked very much, good food and horse back riding. There was a big horse that kicked and a pony and they were called Queenie, Stardust and Cindy. I was glad to see my parents again, so much fun I didn't know what to do. And one special friend I had called Butch. But no one was allowed to cry at that camp, and when I came back I went into my home and it looked just the same, but no one should laugh in my home. Everything seems so small. A few days after I got to my apartment, on August 26th, we decided to go to France. September 11th we sailed on a boat called the 'Liberty'. I was so glad to see Mme Cor again and I had to change my language into French. When I was still in New York I went to a place where there was a nice young lady and it was a kind of school, and if ever I had troubles this lady would help me. She would help me just like Mme Blank does. Mme Blank is really Dougie and her first name is Jimmy, so her real name is Jimmy Durante Dougie McDougall.

But no one knows why if I should sigh. Don't kill me. But if you know why, look at the moon when it shines out and the little crow with thirty branches. Once there was a lady and no horses behind her, and there was a big bug who didn't have any legs, then there was a maid, but she didn't have any head nor any second toe and she cried and cried. Who knows why if I should sigh—don't look down and don't look up. Oh, yes, and now the camera takes me. No no, New York City is pretty and Paris too. But don't say anything for me, for you. I look down, I sigh. Praying gentle James. Three times if you should cry. Praying gentle James. No one knows if you should pose. Oui oui Madame, ne pleurez pas pour moi. Look out and don't say anything. Don't worry if I should sigh. Yes yes yes why not?

There is a marked contrast between the early part of the session where for the first time Sammy talks in a rational way about real past experience and the latter part where he is to a certain extent out of touch with reality. His finding me in the same clothes is reassuring to him. (All his angry feelings have

42

not destroyed me.) But as so often, his positive feelings arouse panic in him, and he appears to let slip in a confused way the distinction between himself and others. His reference to 'Jimmy McDougall and Jimmy Durante' suggests the introduction of a paternal figure into the transference.

13th Session (Saturday 13.11.54)

Sammy demands a glass of water from Hélène, and then tells me that yesterday's story was a true one; he even adds a few details about his life in New York and his journey to Paris. The moment I open my mouth to talk his eyes blaze as though he would like to strike me. He asks me to read out yesterday's story, and while I am reading it he leans across the table and kisses me. From time to time he sings softly and gaily 'the face, the pace, the pretty little face'. He then wants to hear 'Knockerlopp'. He makes various little gestures which seem designed to provoke some reaction from me, such as attempting to knock over a standard lamp. At one point he takes the paint-jar full of water and begins to pour water on the table.

S. – I don't know if I want to or if I don't. Should I? Oh well.

He breaks off and suddenly pours the whole lot onto the table and later manages to tip the table in such a way that the water falls onto the floor. He then dictates the following story:

'The Great Adventure.' Well, however are we going to get this moving, said the young man with the rocket ship. I was planning to take a trip to the moon, but no one knows why the moon is so bright in the sky, and he really made the rocket go. Look out, said a voice, that rocket is going to fall down. So everybody looked out. No, no, said a voice, don't make the rocket go that fast. I turned over on thirty wings and everybody tried to make it go faster. Now it was going higher and higher, but no one knows why. It turned first on one side and then on the other, and went so high it got colder and colder, and at last they landed on the moon. But they'd got it going so fast they couldn't do a thing. But no one knows why. And now we must find things as we turn around the moon three times. They climbed mountains and mountains, thirty hundred of them. Then the man from the rocket ship told the other man what happened to him when he was a little boy. I told my mother I wanted a sweater just like hers, and she said, yes dear, I'll buy you one. So the next day she bought him one just like hers, and he put it on and said it's alright, but it's not like yours, because your sweater has bumps in it. (Sammy turns to me.) My mother told that story to me.

Sammy dictated three more stories in the same vein.

14th Session (Monday 15.11.54)

Sammy asks for 'a little water' this time, and seems upset when I say I shall get it for him since Hélène is not here today.

S. – Well where is she? What's wrong with her?
J. M. – She has a cold. She's just having a rest.
S. – Well, never mind. Let's get on with the story. Oh dear, what shall it be?
J. M. – You don't have to tell stories you know, if you don't want to.
S. – Yes, I *do* want. (He shouts at me.) Get to work!! Take up your pencil, no fooling! Etc.

After searching desperately for ideas he finally recounts a confused version of a film he has seen. I have the feeling that Hélène has acted as a barrier between Sammy and his oral demands towards me, and thus served to lessen his anxiety. He is more dictatorial than ever today and desperate to dominate the situation. (He has, so to speak, lost some magic control in not being able to command Hélène. Perhaps she represents an omnipotently controlled 'breast'.)

At one point in the story there is a dispute between two men about the necessity of killing animals to eat. 'My stomach is sick of killing', says one, and the other replies, 'Don't be a chump, what else can you do, *you must have food*.' The film story deals with 'good' and 'bad' people, and the search for food. Once again before the end Sammy makes everything 'good' and peaceful as though to repair any damage that might have occurred.

15th Session (Tuesday 16.11.54)

From the moment he gets into the consulting-room Sammy shouts commands at me as he did yesterday. He drinks some water out of the paint jar with a grumpy look on his face, then pours the remainder on the floor.

S. – Come along, read out yesterday's story.

I no sooner begin to read than he interrupts me. After every few words he breaks in to say that I am reading too quickly, too slowly, too loudly, too softly, and in addition I have to begin at the beginning every time. Suddenly he begins to shout.

S. – I'm bored, I'm bored—I'm sick of it. There's nothing to do here but to tell stories.

J. M. – You don't have to tell stories.

S. – But there's nothing else for me to do here. (His eyes fall on the paint, plasticine, etc.) I don't want to paint. I don't want to draw, I can't stand coloured crayons. Plasticine, that's boring, and I've got all these things at home. I want checkers and games to play, now!

J. M. – You know we don't have any.

S. – But you should have these things if you want children to come here.

J. M. – Sammy, why do you think children come here?

S. – To talk about things, and *I don't want to.* Now, Dr G., she gave me ice-cream and sweets and had something new every time I went to see her. I loved going there and I always loved coming here but not know.

J. M. – I wonder why you're so afraid of being bored.

S. – Oh, what am I going to do!

The door-bell rings; it is Sammy's mother who is early. Sammy checks this fact by looking at his watch.

S. – Oh, that's mother, but I can't go yet, there's still ten minutes left. That's not fair.

J. M. – But if you're so bored.

S. – Yes, but—we'll see if I can't fill in the last few minutes somehow.

J. M. – You ask me to give you lots of things to eat and new things to play with all the time as if you don't like to have a minute empty.

S. – Well, it's just that I don't know what to do at home now. Dad won't fix the phonograph and I love music. I get so bored at home.

He goes on to describe how he runs to talk with Mme Cor whenever he is bored with his toys. A lady comes to take him out every afternoon and then he is brought here. He gives the impression that every minute of his time is filled in for him; he never has to face the anxiety of being left to do what he chooses.

J. M. – It sounds as if you like to have everything thought out for you, and someone to give you something or do something for you all the time, Sammy?

S. – No, I can do things. But I'm too old for some of my toys.

J. M. – Which ones?

S. – Well, ah, boats and things. . . . It's a worry. I don't know if boats are bad or not. (He looks very worried indeed as he reflects over this question.)

S. – Well, that wasn't so bad, we got over those ten minutes, didn't we?

16th Session (Thursday 17.11.54)

Flings himself into his chair and sighs tragically.

S. – I don't know how I'm going to manage. This is the most boring place I've ever been in. The only place I'm ever bored. Never bored at home. There's that nice Madame Cor who always does something for me, and Ginette who takes me out and Madame Dupont at school.

J. M. – You want me to be like the others and give you games and food and ideas.

S. – Of course you don't have to if you don't *want* to. But it's going to be awful coming here like this. I'll always be bored now.

J. M. – What happens if you get bored?

S. – I told you about that yesterday. Of course, it wouldn't happen if only you had things and ideas for me.

J. M. – You want me to fill up your mind with my thoughts?

S. – But *everybody* does something for me. At home I have so many things, even at school in the morning I have work to do. You can't even do that for me. I only enjoyed coming here because I could tell you stories. Something I can't do at home, but I'm bored with it now. At home I listen to the phonograph when it's not broken. I love drawing but I don't want to here, it would be boring.

J. M. – Even though you love it?

46

S. – Yes, I'd sooner be bored here.

J. M. – I think that's right.

S. – Yes, well, I'd sooner be bored here than at home. Goodness! How am I going to fill in the last half hour? No games, nothing.

J. M. – Perhaps you're a bit afraid of being here with me when we haven't any set games to play.

S. – I'm not, I'm just bored. (He gazes out through the window.)

J. M. – You look as though you would like to run away from me out of this room.

S. — How do you know?

J. M. – Perhaps you feel a bit scared sometimes.

S. – No, I just thought it was going to be nicer.

J. M. – What did you expect?

S. – Well, ah . . . well, new games. But if you haven't got any I'm not asking you to get them.

J. M. – And now you're feeling bored because there's just you and me.

S. – Oh, if you're going to make a conversation . . . ! (He jumps up and starts running around the room with jerky movements like a two year old. He bumps into objects and falls over from time to time. At one moment he catches his jersey with his teeth and pulls at it wildly. He keeps looking at me to see my reactions.)

J. M. – Perhaps you feel like biting your jersey, Sammy, because you're so cross with me.

Sammy continues to fly wildly around the room. I make a little figure in plasticine and begin to talk to it, making things for it to eat and sympathising with its fright. Sammy comes close immediately and listens intently. He takes up the plasticine as though about to join in the game then apparently remembering that he is on strike throws it down again, shouting 'No, I don't want to do it!' After another minute gyrating round the room he comes back to his chair and picks up some plasticine.

S. – I want to make something. This is a head, a real living person. Guess who?

J. M. – You tell me.

S. — It's my sister. I was pretty upset when my mother said she was going to have my baby sister. I wanted to be the only one,

47

but it's different now. I never knew she'd be so cute. She has a funny little nose and a big mouth. She's got the biggest mouth in the world, big as a hippopotamus. (He holds up the head for me to see.) Look out! Your squashing her head. Have you any children? Oh, well, if you don't want to tell me! (He throws the head down on the table.)

S. – (In a loud dramatic voice.) Now I shall kill her. (He stabs the head fiercely with a pencil.) Now she's dead! (Rapidly fashions an elephant.) Look, he's good this elephant. Now he's got to die. Look out! Mind your hands stupid, I might really hurt you. (He stabs the elephant.) Now let's get that lady who looks after the baby, oh yes, the elephant will charge her with his trunk. (He bashes the two plasticine models together.)

The telephone rings in the next room and although I make no move to leave Sammy shouts. 'Oh don't go, please don't go. I want to tell you about this morning. I was very very angry and then the curb got in my way and I fell over it and got hurt.'

J. M. – Perhaps you think things ought to punish you if you get angry.
S. – Oh, no, I don't think the curb really did it. But I'd like to know more about children who *have* thoughts like that. Do they ever get over their problems? What are my problems? Will I get over my problems?

When his mother arrived, Sammy rushed into the waiting-room and said, 'Well, I didn't get so bored after all.'

Sammy continues throughout these two sessions to complain about the frustrations of the analytic situation. He demands either that the analyst treat him like the other adults, that is, as an unpredictable invalid for whom new interests must constantly be found, or that she supply him with oral gifts as he claims his former therapist did.

He obviously feels the loss of the protection the stories afforded him in his attempts to control the transference situation, and in particular the Magic Face anxieties. Perhaps my attempts to discuss the stories have alerted Sammy and made him renounce them as a refuge. The atmosphere changes with the introduction of the plasticine figure. Sammy immediately makes the analyst into the mother who is telling him of her pregnancy. This leads to fantasies of the baby as the result of intercourse which in turn stirs up anxiety and once again we have images of destruction and people getting killed.

It is interesting to see that in the following session he projects onto the *analyst* his wish-fantasy of killing the baby. Sammy now becomes the child that the analyst will leave alone to die.

17th Session (Friday 19.11.54)

Sammy flops into his chair sighing, 'Oh I can't stand being bored' but he smiles at me as though we share a secret joke. I agree that it is a pretty tough situation.

> S. – If I fell out of this window down those three storeys on to the street, you wouldn't even bother to get an ambulance to take me to hospital. You'd just let me die.
>
> J. M. – You really can't count on me at all?
>
> S. – Oh no, You don't *like* me.

He flops back into his chair and continues to talk about his famous boredom. Then he begins running around the room in the same jerky way, coming close to my chair but taking care to avoid any physical contact. As this diffuse activity seems unlikely to abate, I again make a little plasticine boy to whom I address my remarks as though he were Sammy, hoping to provide a medium between himself and me through which he may communicate safely. He joins in with a vivid story about a boy who ran away from his home in Paris, into the woods where he meets an elephant, and at the same time a great 'thing' drops upon the boy from the sky. The Magic Face appears in the air.

> S. – (Breaking off in mid-sentence.) No. I don't want this game. I'm bored. I don't want to talk about him. He's only clay. Me, I'm bored.
>
> J. M. – Maybe you don't want to think about the Magic Face or that thing that dropped from the sky—like your baby sister.
>
> S. – (By now rushing wildly around the room and over the furniture.) Yes, yes. That's it. (He is making such a rumpus

49

that it is surprising he even hears me. He comes across a box of matches which he finds in my desk.) Ha ... let's do experiments! (He lights a match and puts it under the paint-jar from which he had previously drunk all the water.) Now what would you do if the house went on fire? I know. You'd only save yourself, you would!

J. M. – I must say you don't seem to think I can be much help if you're in trouble.

S. – Well if my finger got burned what would you do?

J. M. – I think we'll find out why you have so many worries about what might happen to your body.

For the first time today, Sammy quietens down a little, and till the end of the session plays with the matches. He makes a fuss about leaving and remarks that as long as there are matches to play with he will come back tomorrow.

I am undecided whether to give him matches or not. It seems that if he does not feel loved in the way he wants — with gifts, or as an injured or ill child — the image he has of himself becomes disturbed. He then feels unprotected and expresses this aggressively (but projected onto the angry elephant or the Magic Face).

18th Session (Saturday 20.11.54)

S. – Today, I'm not bored because I know what we're going to do.

J. M. – It seems that when you are able to direct everything you don't have anything to fear from me. Maybe wanting games already prepared is a way of not feeling worried or frightened.

S. – Yeah, that's right! But what about this fire. I don't want to start it yet. Just let's think about it. I know, let's write a story about it first. Come on, get to work. Now just write No No No! Here we are together. This fire is called great burning bitch. And the other was the son of battle. Blup blup blup. Go on, write it all down! Now I shall sing the music for the two fires. Splash splash. The fire is on and out in two minutes. Once there was a lady and that's the end of you poo-poo. No one knows what I shall say what I shall do. But when shall I say something? Nobody knows. That's the end of the story bums.

Sammy demands that his dictation be read back. By then he can wait no longer for his fire. He sticks the few matches which are in the box into the plasticine and lights them with dramatic comments as though he were on stage, then demands more and is furious when I say there are none. He pitches the pencils across the room, picks up the pot of water and hesitates about throwing it too. I don't want water all over the walls, and I tell him this.

S.–But I must throw it. Why can't I do it. I want to get it over with.

He finally lets it trickle very slowly out on to the table.

S.–I want to break something. Which things do you like best?
J. M.–I like all my things, and I don't want them thrown around.
S.–Can I throw this? Or this? Or this?

I tell him that he is trying to provoke me, perhaps in the hope of getting punished, but he will not tolerate the slightest comment. He litters the room with waste-paper rubbish, turns a small table upside down and places my desk lamp on the floor.

S.–Now what do you think?

Without waiting for a reply he darts to the mantelpiece and breaks the two candles. (Where the bull had been in his drawing in session one.)

S.–I feel so strong now. I'm glad I did that.
J. M.–I think I know how you feel. You want to break up the things that you think are important to me. (He stands still for a moment his small face clouded and anxious.) You have not hurt me, Sammy, and I shall not hurt you. We are both quite safe.

Sammy immediately sets about tidying up, singing to himself.

S.–I only did it for some excitement so I wouldn't get bored. I want to tear all your house down. It's the most boring house I know. You won't tell my mother will you? (He has put this question two or three times already and I had told him that I did not talk about our sessions to his parents, though knowing there was little hope that he would believe me.)
J. M.–You seem to think your mother wouldn't approve of what you do here.

S. – What will your husband say?

J. M. – What do you think he'll say?

S. – He'll be so angry he'll kill me. I don't want him to know. He'll get the police after me and I'll get put in jail. Please swing me round.

He drops into my arms saying he can't stand. It is the end of the session and he demands that I carry him into the waiting-room. Since he flatly refuses to budge, I carry him out and set him down before the waiting-room door.

> Sammy's game with fire represents for him a forbidden activity and his 'here we are . . . great burning bitch and the son of battle' suggests a primitive erotic exchange and one for which he later feels impelled to provoke punishment. There are the elements of an oedipal drama here and Sammy is out to get rid of the analyst's husband, but first he must steal his power magically, by breaking the two candles (the symbolic bull of his very first drawings which subsequently makes him 'feel strong'). Little wonder that he then imagines the analyst's husband will kill him for this. As though to say he is too small to have committed the symbolic castration of the father, he play-acts towards the end of the session the small baby whose only relation to the mother-analyst is to be carried around. The session reflects jealousy of the husband probably fantasied as the penis-candle hidden in the analyst!' I want to tear your whole house down.')

19th Session (Monday 22.11.54)

On entering the room, Sammy ransacks my desk for matches. By chance he discovers a small packet of book matches. He bosses me around, telling me to sit still, to be careful not to bump the table, and so on, while he makes a small hump of plasticine into which he sticks the matches and a large coloured pencil. He then orders me to take down the following story:

'This is called Fireworks. Two people in a house lit the fire and it burned and burned as the great blue pencil with a bit of yellow on the top, the tippy top of the clay mountain. The burning matches and the old pencil stayed straight as a tower, point to the ceiling, bottom in the clay. This fire is called great fireworks, and this is the most magnificent fire of all, the best that anyone would see. Eighty times of flame going out and the old pencil still standing. Sparks blew out, three matches more were lit and the flames glittered against the pencil side, and finally one match was left. As it burned against the pencil the fire got smaller. So tiny it looked like an ant with its eyeballs lit. The fire hit the clay. Tock! Out! End of the great fire. No more. Just a bunch of matches. After that Madame McDougall put the clay back, and Mr Sammy went home to his mother.'

Story and fire finished, Sammy immediately shouts at me not to touch the clay mountain, although I have not moved, and am indeed still writing down the end of the story. Sammy makes little menacing gestures towards me with his fists clenched.

     S. – Are you afraid of me?
J. M. – I think it's more likely you who's afraid of me. You keep warning me not to move as though you think I'm dangerous.
     S. – You might knock my head off, or cut me. Or knock my teeth out.
J. M. – That's a load of frightening things. I wonder whether you're afraid you might want to do things to me?
     S. – Well I might kill you and cut off your leg. What would you do then, eh?
J. M. – We'll find out what all these ideas mean one day. I won't let anything too frightening happen to us.
     S. – (Singing.) Oh the face the pace the pretty little face.

Following my interpretation that he is afraid of his projected destructive feelings, in an upsurge of more relaxed positive feeling he gives me a large amorous smile. This disappears shortly after, as though the feelings which accompany his little 'love song' are more troubling than the aggressive interchange. At that moment he recalls that his parents have an appointment to see me this evening.

     S. – Don't tell my parents . . . what *are* you going to tell them tonight? Tell the good things not the bad. My father will come along too. He's stronger than you. He'll bash you up! (He pauses a moment as though contemplating this scene.) What did you husband say about the broken candles?

I hesitate a moment while trying to decide which aspect of this important question to interpret. Sammy jumps up shouting that he is looking for things to break.

J. M. – You know Sammy, it seems to me you're afraid of what will happen if we go on being friendly here together. You wonder what my husband will do about it, and what your mother and your father might think. (It is hard to get a word in, with Sammy flying round the room making loud noises and knocking things over.)

S. – I don't know what might come out of you. I'll kick your stomach out! (He suddenly comes upon a man's pipe.) Ooooh . . . I won't touch anything of his!

J. M. – What would happen?

S. – He'd get the police after me. I'll just touch your things.

J. M. – It seems to me you're frightened of my husband because you and I play games together. But in a way you're even more frightened of me, and that makes you angry with me.

S. – Because you don't give me any games. And I'll go on till you do. Oh, don't tell my parents. You know all my feelings. But you mustn't tell them.

J. M. – You don't trust me, do you?

S. – No. I just don't believe you won't tell them.

The reassurance that nothing harmful will happen produced positive feelings in Sammy and led to some typically oedipal material. But reassuring words are rarely capable of calming the anxiety of a child for whom fantasy is the sole means of apprehending reality. Sammy's regression later in the session suggests that this intervention was rejected.

In an attempt to deal with the oedipal situation Sammy invokes an angry image of the analyst's husband and later fears that his own father will be furious with him too. He protects himself against preodipal fears too (the frightening things inside the analyst) in his recourse to a powerful masculine image. 'My father'll bash you up.' (At the same time he is denying here his own wish to possess his father's power.) Through projective identification he defends himself against his more pregenital fears. He is afraid I will cut him to pieces, but later he is the one who will 'kick my stomach out'. And so on . . .

20th Session (Tuesday 23.11.54)

Today I decided to remove tempting breakable objects since I no longer have confidence that I can confine Sammy to merely verbal expression. He begins kicking at the desk, then my armchair, looking at me covertly after each kick as though waiting for my reaction. He asks for matches and I tell him there are none.

He starts to run aimlessly around the room. His provocative behaviour seems to me a direct consequence of the oedipal guilt-feelings aroused yesterday. I note down what he is doing, and what I think he is expressing, in the hope of being able to interest him later to talk about his feelings. He jumps over a small stool, turns upside down the (empty) wastepaper basket, and says, 'Ah, this is getting really hard'. Switches on the lights, plugs in the standard lamp, shouts one, two, three, go. Pulls off his jersey and throws it on to my lap; puts the plasticine pot on the stool 'to make it a little harder'; bangs into my chair.

> S. – What are you thinking about?
> J. M. – That your parents were here last night to see me.
> S. – Did you tell?
> J. M. – What did you think I would tell them?
> S. – I'm not occupied with that subject at the moment.

He continues running about, then comes over besides me.

> S. – Please, please tell me what you've been writing.

I do so, inserting interpretations as I go, and he listens enraptured. Briefly I tell him that I think he is too upset about all the exciting things in the stories to want to continue with them. Being peaceful here with me seems frightening and he prefers to clown rather than talk. He seems especially worried that my husband will not approve of his thoughts about me. The ideas about kicking out my stomach make him want to kick things around inside my room rather than see what the frightening ideas about my stomach represent.

> S. – Well now I'll get back to my game. Everything will be put back for a happy new year. Just keep on with your letter chum. But you're not right about the stories. You ex- ex- you exaggerate! What did you tell my parents?
> J. M. – You're afraid your father will learn your thoughts and get angry.

S. – Go back to your writing. You can think all you want to but it's not so. I'm not afraid of *anything*. (Sammy sits down beside me and explains in a patient voice.) You see there are lots of people like that. They do a job for a long time and then they get tired of it and they want to go on to another job. It doesn't mean they're afraid of the first job. I just stopped. I didn't have any more ideas.

Having failed to get Sammy talking on the oedipal fears I turn to the pre-oedipal maternal image, and ask whether continuing the ideas might make him think that the Magic Face would really do dreadful things.

S. – Yes . . . but . . . no, no. I'll write some stories another time.

Sammy goes off calmly. For the first time in a week he says good-bye and gives me a big smile.

21st Session (Thursday 25.11.54)

S. – I'm not afraid about the stories, because I'm not afraid of anything.

J. M. – So you feel I'm wrong about this?

S. – And I don't want any conversations . . . see!

He starts to jump over things and throw paper around.

J. M. – You want to throw things about and jump around rather than talk to me. But it's another way of telling me things too.

S. – I don't want to discuss that subject. I wanted matches, and things to play with. Now I'm going to do this instead. And stop talking.

J. M. – Afraid of what I'm going to say?

S. – Don't talk! If you do I'll . . . well you'll see.

J. M. – I can understand that it makes you angry that I just talk and don't have lots of games and so on to fill up the time.

S. – Yes! Now stop talking or I'll . . . (he holds up his fist).

J. M. – What will happen?

Sammy gets up and with great dignity walks out of the room. I see his small shadow which indicates that he is peeping through the crack of the door. I say out loud, 'Sammy would just like to give me a hit because of all the bothering ideas that come up here. He would like to punish me, but he also wanted to protect me, so he decided to run out of the room instead. I don't give him lots of things to play with and things to eat like the other people, and that makes him angry.' Sammy comes suddenly back into the room and glaring at me says:

S. – Did you just not get any matches because you know I enjoy them *so much*?

J. M. – So you think I want to forbid you doing exciting things here with me?

S. – Well . . . if you had some games . . . but I suppose you wouldn't spend the money. You're mean. You don't give me anything at all.

J. M. – You think I don't like you because I don't give you all the things you would like?

S. – No, it's the other way round. I don't like anybody who doesn't give me all the things I want and doesn't do things for me!

J. M. – The others do things to stop you getting bored?

S. – You just *want* me to get bored. And if I like something very much you'll take it away. Couldn't we even have matches?

J. M. – Well, I'll think about it.

22nd Session (Friday 26.11.54)

In the hope of getting some of Sammy's fire fantasy into the sessions I decided to put out a box with a few matches in it. He is very excited to find them. He places half of them into a ball of plasticine and says he will make a story about it first, which at his request I note down.

'Now this fire is going to start. And the best fire of all. The fire which I've been wishing for, for days and days. And I never know yet what to think. I never never had so much fun in all my life. (He lights some matches.) And then all the fire went out. But it doesn't matter. That's there for good. And the next day will be some more. That's all, bums! (He now lights the remaining matches.) Now we have a big firework like the 14th July. Our fire is a magic fire, the best anyone has ever seen. It's name is Pisa, after the leaning tower that no one has ever seen. Ever seen such a fire. The best, never the worst.'

Sammy asks me three different times if I like the fire.

J. M. – Were you afraid I wouldn't?

    S. – Don't start this afraid business again! Now let's get this straight about what I really like to do.

J. M. – O.K. let's get it straight.

    S. – Now you take down the things I like doing best.

> *Best Things*: Games
> Eating ice cream
> Having interesting conversations
> Having fire in the fireplace
> Classical music
> Candles
> Paintings by Matisse and Rembrandt
> Tempera paint
> Drawings

Now write down the worst things I like.

> *Worst things*: Being bored
> Talking about things
> Jumping over wastepaper baskets
> Playing uninteresting games I don't know how to play
> Baby records and ugly music

Sammy then constructs a composite list of all possible activities in order of preference.

1. Games. 2. Ice cream. 3. Big matchbox and candles. 4. Interesting conversations about what I do during the day and in the weekends. 5. Making things out of modelling clay. 6. Writing stories. 7. Painting with watercolours. 8. Jumping over chairs and baskets. 9. Talking about when I'm afraid and things I don't like. 10. Being bored and having nothing to do.

23rd Session (Saturday 27.11.54)

I have a bad cold which is obvious the moment I say good-day to Sammy.

    S. – (In an accusing voice.) You're sick!

He sits down and begins to mould bits of plasticine and asks if he can add to yesterday's tower. He talks briefly about his horse-riding exploits, and I am surprised to hear him talk for once about some outer events. He is looking at me apprehensively, and I get the impression he is talking distractedly. He becomes more and more restless, and a slow note of panic creeps into his voice, till he suddenly breaks off.

S. – Get back, get back you. You got a cold! I might get your cold. You're bad. You smell bad. Why didn't you 'phone me. You have no right to see me when you have a cold!!

J. M. – You think I might be dangerous to you, that what comes out of me might harm you?

S. – (His panic mounting.) Don't talk! Don't breathe at me!! (I am at this point more than three feet away. He shoves the plastic plasticine jar towards me.) Here, put this over your mouth!

I do so without comment (after debating whether to interpret his contamination fears and their relation to his own aggressive desires and his fear that they might come back out of my mouth).

S. – Now keep it there and don't talk.

Then follows a stream of abuse and bizarre threats of every kind, of which I noted a small sample after the session.

S. – You'll be punished for this . . . I'll slap your ears down. You'll be sorry you done it . . . I'll slap your bottom off. I'll tear your behind off. You'll be sorry . . . etc.

His little face contorted with rage and fright, he begins to scream.

S. – Don't talk! Don't move!! (I haven't moved an inch during his long outburst.)

Sammy continues in this fashion for almost 15 minutes, and sometimes sounds just like an angry parent admonishing a child.

S. – I've had enough of you, do you hear? Now that'll do! One more word out of you . . . and you'll be sorry. Not a word. Stop talking I say! (He looks at me, immobile behind my plasticine pot.) Stop moving! The fingers of your left hand are moving. Stop it now. Don't *breathe* so much. I can hear you breathing! You'll be punished. Oh I'll slap your behind

right off. I've had enough of you. I'll cut your mouth off. I've
You'll be punished. You won't have any *fire*!!

During this tirade he prepares his fire, and then proceeds to place
the whole structure ready for lighting on the brass table which is
between our two chairs. Although this isn't very dangerous I had
forbidden it in earlier sessions stipulating that matches could only be
lit in the fireplace. He has been inciting me in sado-masochistic
fashion to talk, by daring me not to, and I felt that this was another
such ploy. I come out at this point from behind my pot.

J. M. – No Sammy! You may only light the fire in the fireplace
      otherwise I shall have to take the matches.
  S. – (Rushing forward to light his fire mountain rapidly.) No.
      Now, now. Stop it you!
J. M. – Don't be a silly boy.

Sammy sulkily moves his structure over to the chimney place.

  S. – Now get back and don't say things!!

He lights his fire reserving a few matches, and then throws on all
the drawing paper he can find. He prepares to throw the crayons and
the box, which I forbid.

  S. – Keep quiet you . . . I'll cut you up, your mouth, your bot-
      tom . . . You got a cold, and you're going to be punished. Oh
      you're so bad tempered today, and you don't even know it.
J. M. – I think it's you who's feeling bad tempered.
  S. – But not as bad as you are (he springs up in sudden panic).
      Oh you won't tell my mother will you? Answer me, answer
      me!
J. M. – What are you scared your mother will find out?
  S. – Tell me. Will you? Will you?
J. M. – You think we're doing something naughty here that your
      mother wouldn't like?
  S. – (Pointing to the fire.) This? Yes. Don't you? Oh you won't
      tell will you or I'll get punished (he jumps madly up and
      down).
J. M. – I don't tell your parents what you do in your sessions. But I'm
      sure you think that playing with matches and fire is some-
      thing like what adults—your mummy and daddy—do when
      the children aren't around. And that's why you think she will

be cross. As if you are playing a game with me like dad might play with your mother.

S. – (Suddenly calm again.) Yes!! So you see, you won't tell will you?

He makes a great fuss about leaving at the end of the hour. When his mother arrives to collect him he says pointedly in front of her to me, 'Will you get some more matches for Wednesday?'

J. M. – Wednesday is the day you don't come to see me.

S. – Yes, but Thursday, not Monday though. Oh get them Monday, Tuesday or Wednesday.

Added to the idea that words in themselves are dangerous there is today the emergence of oral contamination fears, and these stimulate in Sammy fantasies of anal-sadistic revenge. In his desire to 'slap my bottom off' he is no doubt identifying with his mother when he provoked her into slapping him. A forbidden erotic relationship is thus re-enacted accompanied by appropriate punishment. Sammy accepts the interpretation that the fire game is linked with the primal scene, but he is then forced to display this to his mother after the session. His guilt and anxiety make him confused about which days he comes to sessions.

24th Session (Monday 29.11.54)

Sammy is fifteen minutes late. He had refused to leave the ice rink when Ginette called him. She said just two more rounds and he had done eighteen.

J. M. – I guess you didn't want to come here today.

S. – Yes, I didn't want to. There's nothing to do.

J. M. – Maybe also it was because of our fire game?

S. – This place is no good. No games, no matches, nothing, and I don't want the sort of games you mean, games we make up and play together. No thank you! Not me!

J. M. – You don't think it's safe for us to play games together?

S. – Now that's enough of that. I don't want any of your conversations.

61

He starts running around knocking things over, apparently deaf to any remarks I make. 'This is a hateful place. It's so awful I just mighn't come back.' He then comes and sits down again. He tells me that he doesn't like knocking things over but that he doesn't know what else to do. I take advantage of this moment of calm to tell him that I understand how he feels, and how difficult it is for him with no set games.

> S. – That lady in New York, she gave me ice cream and toy soldiers. But you don't even give me a box of matches. I'd be happy with the cheapest most ordinary game. What I really want is chess, but since you don't have that . . . You know what I'd really like is the phonograph, and chess and painting with oils (this latter is not allowed by his father at home) but since you don't have them . . . well. (Sammy throws a glance at the phonograph which is in the corner of the room, and which he always avoids as though it were taboo.)
> S. – Would you get me a game? Just some little thing and I'd play and play and be happy. Oh you wouldn't. (Without the barrier of games he feels that the contact is too close and he is at the mercy of his impulses.)

J. M. – You think I don't protect you from the bad things that happen when children get bored?

Sammy was very agitated during this conversation and had hardly let a moment elapse without throwing things or shouting at me to shut up. But for an instant he becomes calm.

> S. – Well would it be alright to have games?

J. M. – I'll see. But we should also try to understand why you're so upset when there aren't any games.

Sammy passed the rest of the session shouting and screaming, a mixture of rage and panic, and I felt completely helpless in my desire to bring him some peace of mind, or to stem the tide of his mounting destructiveness.

> That evening in an attempt to organise my thoughts about him, I noted the following points:
> 1. It seems to me that Sammy cannot support analysis at present without certain direct gratifications, in spite of the complications which this will invariably introduce into the

analysis. (He continues to order milk from Hélène about two times out of three, and also frequently helps himself to the paint water.)

2. I have presumed too much on his intermittent analytic therapy in the past. He has no real acceptance of psycho-analysis as something which might help him with his grave and frightening problems. Analysis and the analyst are something against which he must defend himself at all costs. His mother however has reported that he loves coming and looks forward eagerly to the sessions.

3. He is manifestly terrified of what might happen to him (or me) if we don't have structured games.

4. He has no ability to project his fantasies into games as normal and neurotic children do. The fantasies have some-thing of the omnipotent and cosmically disastrous about them and cannot be readily expressed in terms of play. His mother has always noted that he is quite unable to play either alone or with others.

5. There may be a conflict of loyalties between his New York therapist and me. Dr G was 'good' and he needs to keep her this way.

6. He has an urgent need to control everything, and cannot relax for fear that the relationship will get out of hand. He is immediately flooded with anxiety and terror which he tries to deal with by some form of motor discharge.

7. I feel my interpretations are getting nowhere, and Sammy gets more destructive every day.

8. A new plan of approach seems necessary. Perhaps small figures and animals, such as tiny children play with. He is such a strange and isolated little boy, and perhaps he needs to play back at the level of a three- or four-year-old. Will throw out the coloured crayons which he keeps telling me he hates. Games for him mean chess—his one achievement in the field of play. His parents' attempts to interest him in any other games have proved futile. I could bring out the chess set. I don't want to run the risk of interfering with this activity which is valuable in his relationship with his father. There are always the 'forbidden' matches. These probably represent masturbation and primal scene fantasies and also a way of discharging and controlling destructive wishes.

25th Session (Tuesday 30.11.54)

Carrying out my new plan of approach I have collected a number of plastic toys, including people, wild and domestic animals, a baby, a policeman, a pram and an ambulance. I also put out a chess set, a box of ordinary lead pencils and paper as usual.

S.–Oh, did you do this for me? Oh I'm so happy. Well I never thought you'd do a thing for me. But supposing—mind it isn't true—I'll never be bored now—but just *supposing* I still get bored with all these things? But I won't, you know.

J. M.–You might, I know.

S.–Well what would you say.

J. M.–I suppose it would mean that you'd rather be bored than play with the things, that it isn't really games you want. It would be a way of telling me something, and we would try to find out together just what it was, and what you are really searching for.

S.–Oh I won't get bored. But if I did—if I wanted something— let me see—what if I wanted something else?

J. M.–What might it be?

S.–Well I might want an apartment, exactly like this one, all for myself. What would you say?

J. M.–Then I'd think that you wanted to live with me—in my apartment.

S.–(Laughs.) Oh boy! Now what shall I play with? Let's leave the chess aside. (He picks up the box of plastic toys.) I wonder why you took so long to get them.

J. M.–I began to understand how uncomfortable you felt when there were no toys.

S.–Did you have to pay money for them? Do other children come here? I never see any, only some big people. Do other children play alone here like you and me? What do you do with the big people? Etc. etc. (He does not seem to mind, for once, not having his questions answered, and is meanwhile sorting out the animals and the male figures, soldier, farmer, policeman. Back into the box go all the female figures, pram, baby and ambulance.) Shall we have a story? Here you tell me a story.

J. M.–What do you suggest?

S.–Well this is a game of three good people and three bad people. The good people are hungry. They go out to catch a giraffe to

64

eat. The people then get eaten by a tiger. (At this point Sammy takes a rhinoceros which begins charging and knocks down good and bad people alike—as though unable to differentiate the good and bad fantasies attached to phallic expressions.)

S.—It's a pity you haven't a hippo. But never mind. I won't ask you to get anything else. That will do for that. (He puts all the toys away in the box.) Let's play chess.

Sammy sets up the pieces, and allows me to choose for colours with my eyes closed. He is quite upset that I choose white. He also expresses disappointment that I already know how to play. We play for about twenty minutes and I win narrowly. (It should perhaps be noted that I play chess rather badly, and that in my game with Sammy I was doing my best.) He demands that we replay the ending. He gets a pawn onto my back line in this revised version of the game, and takes my white queen instead of his own to replace it. He is astounded when I point out his error. At the end of the session he strongly resists going home, but finally leaves singing 'The face the pace the pretty little face.'

> When Sammy threatens to get bored even with the longed-for toys he implicitly acknowledges that he is in no way protected from the dangerous libidinal and aggressive relationship he fears between us. However, he does proclaim his desire to have everything (including the analyst and the apartment) so that he manages for a moment to deny the anxieties connected with oedipal fantasy and even more frightening preoedipal fears of total destruction.

> It is interesting to note that his game concerns primitive eating fantasies—the tiger eats up the family who have found themselves a giraffe to eat. (Incorporation of the paternal phallus brings death from the devouring mother tiger.) At the end of the session Sammy needs me to play chess with him as his father does, perhaps as a protection against the frightening mother image.

26th Session (Thursday 2.11.54)

Sammy again expresses his pleasure in the toys and asks me why I had got them for him.

I repeat my former explanation.

    S. – Oh you've got a hippo! Oh lovely. And there's that cow. Now you write!

Now this cow (he relates rather than plays) could not bear anyone near him. He gets so nervous when people come near that he kicks. This makes the others attack him. It's really the cow's own fault, but he thought it was the fault of the others. Then all the wild animals surround the cow, and the hippo is pushed forward to bite off his tail. (This bit of the drama is enacted.) The cow is now too frightened to do anything so it just goes along with the others. (Sammy fishes the kangaroo out of the box, saying it is a friendly animal, and can't be put with the others. Indeed, apart from the cow, he has not as yet showed any interest in the 'friendly' domestic animals.) Now there's a big fire in the forest. (He begins to get very excited, and attempts to make the fire spread beyond the confines of the chimney-place, and is furious when I prevent this. He quietens down when I continue to give help with the 'forest fire'.

    S. – Were you scared of the fire?

J. M. – No, but I don't want my things to get burned.

Whereupon Sammy seizes the rest of the papers on the table and throws them into the remnants of the fire, followed by the matchbox and a few pencils, which don't burn up too well. He then lunges suddenly to the plasticine and throws lumps of it round the room.

    S. – Now how do you like that? What else can I break?

He gathers up the pram, doll's bed, ambulance, red truck, smashes them to pieces under his feet and throws them into the fireplace.

    S. – Do you like that?

J. M. – I got them for you so it's up to you what you do with them. I notice that you have smashed up the baby things.

    S. – And the baby! And the silly old mother! (These are smashed up in their turn.) Now we shall have a game of chess.

J. M. – I'm sorry Sammy. There's no time left for today.

    S. – You will! You will! (He taps me on the head with two chess pieces, then turns to the board and picks up the white king.) And this is going to be the *queen*. I don't care what you say. (He gets angry as I quietly pack up, and makes several

66

attempts to hit me which I prevent by ducking out of the way.) Are you crying now?

J. M. – No. But I don't want to be hit.

S. – Why don't you want to be hit?

J. M. – Because I like myself and I don't like being hit.

At that moment Sammy drops one of the chess pieces near my chair and asks me if I will pick it up so he can put it away. I immediately bend down to pick it up, and he gives me a terrific crack on the head with another piece he had hidden in his hand. Under the impact of the pain, I straighten up and am on the point of slapping him. But seeing his face full of hatred mingled with terror, I put my arm round his shoulders and draw him towards me; I give him a mock spank and say, 'Oh you are a scallywag.' He immediately gives a friendly grin.

S. – What's a scallywag?

J. M. – Well it's someone who wants to get close to people, but he's too scared. So he plays little tricks like you did just now so he can do so safely.

S. – (Beaming.) Scallywag! I'm a scallywag!

He leaves very quietly and seems quite reassured.

> Sammy's ambivalence about the toys is evident, but he does allow himself one brief game in which he obviously identifies with the nervous cow. In this same sequence the hippo, (who has already been used in the stories as a pregnant mother-image) punishes him orally. Perhaps this primitive castrative fantasy impels Sammy towards the 'forbidden' fire game once more—to prove that he is very much alive and dangerous. After burning up the mother and the baby he seeks through the chess game some contact with the father, and declares that 'the king shall be queen'. It was probably the frustration of this urgent need that made Sammy attack me physically. He is also scared of his positive feelings. They are probably expressed in the 'forest fire', and also make the end of the session harder for Sammy to tolerate.

27th Session (Friday 3.12.54)

The Brown Cow is again the leading character. In every relationship with the other animals she is clearly 'maladjusted', causing herself to be disliked, principally because she can tolerate nobody near her.

S. – Please write 'Sammy's Game' and put in my ideas.

This is a farm for wild animals as well as others. Brown Cow is here too. He's really quite nice. He only kicks because the others bother him. The charging rhino makes a terrible noise, and then the Brown Cow comes and kicks him. Didn't like him being so close. Now all the animals are back in the farm. It's all safe now. Cow looks around and doesn't care for the two horses beside him, although they never meant to hurt him. The second horse rubs the first one on its side. Brown Cow doesn't join in any of the animals' fun. He is quite alone. He doesn't like all this motionage. All the animals are in peace. The rhino breaks his cage and is going to ruin all the other animals. The little calf comes up to the mother cow, who doesn't want to kick now. (Note the cow has changed sex. She is also a mother.) Cow starts to get excited and trots around all the other animals. They all play now in fun. She kicks the horse, but it is just play. This horse and cow begin to fight, and kick each other very fiercely standing on their hind legs. They both fall over and now, up, they start again. (Sammy repeats three times this suggestive scene.) Now they are all back in the farm where everything is safe.

Sammy is particularly pleased with the ending of his story where security and peace finally reign. He asks if it is possible to have two more cows and another horse. Since it is clear that the cow is playing a double, or confused sexual role, in which not only Sammy himself is represented, but also the mother under her double aspect of feeding the little calf, and having 'fighting-fun' with the horse-father, I promise Sammy that I will get other cows.

Sammy asks me to read back his story 'putting in the thoughts' that is interpretations of the sexual and aggressive themes. I interpret his own anxiety about getting too close to people, but do not touch the material which concerns his unconscious identification with what he feels are his mother's attitudes to him and to the father.

28th Session (Saturday 4.12.54)

Sammy shrieks with delight at finding a new black cow.

S. – Dougie, just write down the story. Not the words but the real thoughts behind it.

Without waiting for a reply he picks up a horse and Brown Cow and stages a particularly sadistic fight between them.

S. – Now what are my thoughts?

J. M. – Well no one can read your thoughts but we can try to work them out, and see what you think. The last time I wrote down some 'real thoughts' it was about mother and dad when they are alone at night. I just wonder if this horse and cow game isn't your idea of what adults do together sexually.

S. – Now let's have another game. Write down the thoughts *please*.

I take down Sammy's words and insert in parenthesis possible interpretations to give him at the end, when reading the story back.

'Black Cow and Wild Horse . . . kick! Kicks! Horse and little Brown Cow get on better together (maybe Sammy is little Brown Cow, and Wild Horse and Black Cow are mummy and daddy. Sammy-Brown-Cow, thinks Daddy-Horse can protect him. He feels lonely and sad, and kicks all the others because he is afraid. It's just his way of protecting himself.) There goes Wild Horse and Black Cow again. They're having a good big kicking fight, a terrible fight and Wild Horse wins. (That's daddy horse and mummy cow, and this is what Sammy thinks they do together. Now he has laid them far apart. I guess sometimes he would like to separate them, and stop them having those games.) Wild Horse and Black Cow are far apart now, and little Brown Cow is getting kicked over to big Black Cow. Write down all my thoughts Dougie. The wild animals are a nice peaceful family. Now try the horses together. There they are, fighting on their high knee-legs. Now put them far apart. Now all the bad family are gone. The good people who don't hurt each other come along (the 'good people' are people who don't play these exciting sexual games). There's trouble ahead because these cows and horses are back. Black Cow hears her baby crying. (Sammy sometimes wants his mother all to himself.) And the cows shouldn't be so bad, so bad together.'

S. – (Looking up from his game.) You know sometimes it's just because they don't know each other they're so afraid and bad.

J. M. – A bit like you and me?

S. – (His face lights up as though he has just understood.) Was I afraid? Yes, I think I was once.

He asks me to read the story back, which I do, inserting the interpretations already noted in parenthesis. He listens with fixed attention.

S.–Please let's have another one (he knows it is the end of the session). Please, please, one where the horse kicks the cow.

J. M.–You want to hear me say again the bit about what the adults do together. But there's no more time.

S.–Ah, the old cow's had enough for today!

J. M.–I guess that Black Cow stands partly for me and partly for your mother.

29th Session (Monday 6.12.54)

S.–Now get down my thoughts because today's story is going to be about Magic Face and about this little horse. It's called Flicker.

And old Magic Face can turn Flicker into all sorts of things and all kind of animals. (Magic Face is me and Flicker is Sammy I think.) Now Flicker finds himself next to Black Cow, and the fight starts with the two cows. There they go and Flicker too. Now they must all go into their stable and be tied together. (This is Sammy-Flicker with mummy cow and daddy-cow. Sammy thinks they'd better get tied. He doesn't want anyone to get hurt in these games.) There they go again. (Here follows a series of kicking fights between different pairs of animals, where one or the other invariably gets kicked on the bottom, or poke their legs, trunks etc., at other animals' bottoms. I put in parenthesis that Sammy is interested apparently in what happens to people's bottoms.) Now all the friends are together. And in comes Flicker. He gets very mad, and kicks and thunders. He's just yelling, and all the animals come out after him. The elephant puts his trunk in Flicker's back leg. Ha! His front foot's fall off!

S.–(Looking up from his game at me.) Just write the idea what I'm thinking. (Sammy is afraid if he joins in the wild games of the mothers and fathers, he will get his own body damaged or broken.)

Now all the animals come to Flicker because he gets so angry. They all bite him. Giraffe paws Flicker's behind, and even the kangaroo tries to hurt him. It's because he kicked. But the little calf stays over here with its mother and helps to get all this badness away (one part of Sammy wants to join in the exciting games, like his father but the other part wants to be protected by his mummy, like the little calf). All the people have come to see what's up. Now Flicker falls down. Sick with tetanus. He's hot all over, and the animals all chase him. Now the animals are being put back, and Flicker is left alone in a corner. (Sammy feels he is so bad that everyone must leave him alone.) Now please write down all my thoughts.

I read back the story and 'thoughts' and Sammy manifests great delight. One 'thought' which I do not give Sammy is that Flicker falls down sick with tetanus after joining his mother. Contact with the pre-oedipal mother-image is physically dangerous. Each time I make the slightest movement Sammy screams at me. I must only write— and here too he controls my pen through his dictation.

30th Session (Tuesday 7.12.54)

I again put interpretations in parenthesis for reading out at the end, since Sammy demands this each time.

> S. – All the horses and cows are in the farm together. They have games, but just little kicks and things . . . etc. (I think Sammy doesn't want them to have as much excitement as yesterday. He thinks like Flicker, that his own body will get damaged if he plays with it, or thinks about what the grown-ups do.)

After a series of similar games he pulls out the chess then puts it back.)

> S. – No! Let's have matches. The Magic Face will do a trick. (He pulls out a Magic Face which he had drawn on paper yesterday.) Three matches said this face with a fairly good smile, and she lights them by magic. Write what I'm thinking. Careful everyone! (Sammy thinks his thoughts are dangerous. He would like to play chess games like with his father. He thinks it might be better than being alone with Dougie-Magic Face.) We'll have a fire to make an exciting ending. You're gonna be punished you are. Here, put Magic Face in the fire. (He turns round several times and menaces me with his fists clenched.) Scallywag. You scallywag.

31st Session (Thursday 9.12.54)

Today Sammy starts off by asking if he could read the stories he wrote 'in those days when I was bored'. He asks me if I remember, as though it were very far in the past. His delight in his stories is immense and he accepts with interest my interpretations about dangerous interchanges. He makes various comments like, 'Oh yes, I used to believe in bad, bad people—when I was a little boy.' Throughout the session he chats freely in somewhat intellectual fashion about himself at the time of dictating the stories. Towards the end of the session when he notices that time is slipping away he immediately wants to start a story game. Since I have the feeling that he wants to take some distance from all the material of the last few sessions, I tell him that there isn't really time to write down the stories and all the thoughts (which he accepts readily), but that he can play a quick game. Black Cow and Bull together kick Wild Horse, then continue their usual games.

This time, on going into the waiting-room, Sammy discovers his father has come to collect him.

S. – Oh, but *you* mustn't come in here.

He looks guilty and agitated, and his whole attitude is quite different from that which he habitually shows when it is his mother who comes.

32nd Session (Friday 10.12.54)

Sammy is in a state of elation throughout this session. He comes in singing. (He never at any time sings any words. Most of the themes are from symphonies he has in his record collection.) He lifts Flicker out of the box and marches him forward singing loudly a theme from the Tchaikovsky's 6th Symphony. Then a horse with a rider on its back is marched in grandiose fashion to loud chanting of a Beethoven theme. Sammy acts like an impresario who is announcing that something exciting is about to happen. The cows are then marched out to an accompaniment of themes from the Pastoral Symphony. A policeman, trees and a second horse are lined up at the back. Sammy stands back and sings in operatic style the Beethoven 'Hymn of Joy'.

S. – Everyone is to follow the Wild Horse (not Flicker) because the man said so. They all go through the wild woods, all the people with troubles. They don't kick, they bite off the leaves which seem good to them. They go through the woods like a knife cutting through bread (the theme song is now Mozart). This policeman is shaking from a heart attack. (Sammy agitates him violently and then pushes him over.) A second man says, 'I'll take care of you all.' Wild Horse kicks Black Cow but the man gives a shout to stop the fighting. Flicker kicks Bull. Here comes Brown Cow. Queenie the Evil One, we call her, because she kicks so hard. She kicks Bull over the cliff, but he's alright and he just manages not to fall over. Now he bucks Queenie. Into her behind! Into her stomach! Into her udder! Queenie kicks back every time. (Sammy sings lustily the theme of 'Wagon Wheels Carry me Home'.) Flicker rears to see what's going on, and Black Cow is nervous too. (Bull, Brown Cow and Queenie have been placed side by side.) Flicker and Black Cow are now friends and they rub noses. (He sings a light, airy theme.) Look now, Bull got a bit jealous of Flicker and Black Cow. So Flicker kicks that other Bull away. (I note interpretation for later on, of Sammy-Flicker's wish to have Dougie-Black Cow's help to face the worries of what Father-Bull and Mother-Brown Cow do together, and of Sammy-Flicker's wish sometimes to kick Dad away. Also he might have thought yesterday when his father came here, that he would be jealous, like Bull in this story.) Flicker trots along and wonders what Black Cow is thinking. (Interpretation that Black Cow is needed but also felt to be pretty dangerous.) This baby calf, he's bored, so bored he doesn't know what to do. Boy is he nervous! He wants to kick but he says 'Well it's just because I'm so nervous and I mustn't kick'. (This is another part of Sammy that isn't sure how he feels about me or about his mummy. Sometimes he wants us to protect him against his bad feelings but at other times he feels we are the bad ones.) Brown Cow finds her calf and it's not bored any more. Flicker leaves Black Cow and goes over to be with Bull. (Sammy can either go back and be protected by Mother or join forces with Father.) People this is the end of the story.

S. – (To me) I was going to play chess but I've thought of something else very exciting. Please write, Dougie.

This is the great day of the horse race (sings theme song 'Barber of Seville'). Horses and cows line up line up! First Bull now Flicker. Wild Horse comes ahead but now he's tired, then Queenie, now Black Cow. It's a close race. Wild Horse is jumping. Flicker lets them go ahead. If he does it too fast he'll be tired at the end. Who's the winner? It's Flicker! He's boiling with sweat and drinking warm water. Flicker's legs are broken, so no one knew he could be so good. The swellest! And it hurt him too. He's overworked himself and now he has to lie down. Everyone comes and pats and licks him. Even though he was bad to them. And all the animals go to different trees to eat. The end.

> The theme seems to be an affirmation of oedipal rivalry and the triumph over castration anxiety. There is a clear progression from the rather crazy oedipal themes of the early sessions to this normal-neurotic oedipal theme. My obvious interest in the intercourse games and fantasies has helped Sammy I think to accept them too. There is even a hint of genital-level affection and forgiveness. Everyone pats and licks Flicker 'even though he was bad', and at the end there's enough for everybody to eat. This is a change from earlier sessions where one had to kill if one wanted to eat.

33rd Session (Saturday 18.12.54)

Today Sammy arrives twenty minutes late, and gives no explanation. He picks up the box of toys then pushes it away saying, 'No. We'll play chess.' He is very quiet and talks in normal, reasonable tones. (Usually his speech is punctuated with squeaks and cries of various kinds.)

S. – Today I want you to teach me all the tricks of chess.

We play and I win the game by a narrow margin. Sammy expresses disappointment, but it is within normal limits, much as any ten-year-old would express himself, and in marked contrast to his reaction to our last chess game.

S. – Dougie, you really are very clever!

> I have the feeling that yesterday's game may have troubled Sammy because of its triumphant theme. In any case he makes it clear that today his friendly relationship with his father is to come to the fore. He is even reassured when I win at chess.

Sammy is again very late, but this time wants to start immediately to play with the box of toys. He picks up the Black Cow.

S. – The Cow. Oh, the Black Cow! What can this story be? Darned if I know. (He looks mysterious and peers at the cow in his hands.) This is getting rather difficult. I can't think of an idea. Even if I had new animals I wouldn't think of much. The new ones wouldn't help. (Looking at me.) It might get boring, but maybe not. I hope it doesn't. Now write down the words and the thoughts! (He begins to sing and line up horses and cows, but doesn't designate which ones are acting.)

There is one cow who doesn't care for the others. He would *do* it any time. Then Wild Horse kicks. And now Flicker kicks Wild Horse. And here's our famous Black Cow. (He holds her high up in the air.) Now the little calf comes and drinks out of the wrong cow. (Calf drinks from Dougie-Black Cow), and Black Cow turns and kicks that calf. Brown Mother-Cow gives three good hard kicks to Black Cow (the two cow mothers). Black Cow said she kicked for a reason. Mother Cow goes to her calf who is very, very sick. And Black Cow bucks at a rock. (Sammy places Mother Cow with two front legs over her calf.) The calf was surprised that the Black Cow kicked because he thought it was his mother, and Mother Cow warns him against Black Cow. Black Cow is so awful she says. Bull is alright, because he's a friend of Mother Cow. Now Bull hates Black Cow, and Flicker comes over and kicks Black Cow. He's a relation of the Black Cow. He can be the father—no, the grandfather. Bull is as happy as can be, and then up comes Black Cow and kicks and breaks his bones. (Dougie is dangerous to Bull-Father.) Then Bull rears and bumps its big behind on Mother Cow. A really bad Bull, bully black Bull, and would kick the ones that are younger than it, too. Now Mother Cow kicks Bull with its big bully behind. The little calf wanders and comes to the Black Cow, and Black Cow kicks out, very savage. This calf, for the Bull's and the Cow's information, the other Cow is trying to get. (Fantasies concerning Sammy, myself, his father and mother. I am a bad mother, and the other is a good one.) Now the Black Cow is bleeding and is out of joint in its back legs. So it went to the doctor, and he took care of it. But no one could take care of the little calf. But he felt wonderful. He feels wonderful, says this Brown Mother Cow, with a little bit of sadness in her voice. For the calf is feeling well in a way that no one cares for. Mother Cow isn't pleased. Bull and the others go over to see the calf. They don't know what is wrong. Mother Cow went away. Now they know the reason. The information shall be found out for you. (Sammy looks at me.) Everyone's gayfulness is away. That nice little calf was *killed* by the Black Cow's kick. For our information—that little calf died!! Now it's in its grave. Mother Cow is not happy at all, she cries beside the little calf. Bull is the calf's uncle and he feels very sorry. (Sammy begins to sing.) Now Little Calf rises up in the air. Everyone is looking at the miracle. Bull suffers to see this bad thing happening. He sees a face in the sky, it goes higher and higher and disappears in the sky. It floats so nicely up to heaven. For it did die. All the animals walk sadly. Mother Cow comes out and is going to fight Black Cow for killing its calf. (Sings tune from Beethoven's 9th.) She fights and kicks and she bites. Bull and Mother Cow both fight Black Cow. Now Black Cow is . . . ah . . . let's see . . . well she's tired . . . ah, and well, she goes home and feels sorry. She's that intelligent. She knows she did something wrong. Bull and Mother Cow since they are relations they talk. Now here's Flicker. He's the father—no—he's the husband of the Mother Cow. Flicker talks to Bull. It's his . . . ah . . . his nephew-in-law. They canter home for fun.

As it is late, I tell Sammy that the story can't be read back with the thoughts which he reclaims, but that we can do that tomorrow.

I note interpretation concerning different aspects of the mother image, and transference aspect of Dougie-Black Cow and Sammy-Calf, against which Bull-father is to protect him. (The death of Little Calf is perhaps the loss of Sammy's baby-self, which Mother wanted to keep but which is menaced by Dougie-Black Cow.)

35th Session (Tuesday 21.12.54)

> S.–Now read my story. (I have no sooner started to read than he interrupts with, 'Don't read it as though you are in love with your husband!')

I give the interpretations of myself as bad Black Cow, a mean kind of mother that it would be dangerous to love. Sammy feels like the little calf and imagines he can get his own back on everyone by dying and making the others very sad. But it is perhaps a baby-part of himself which has died.

> S. – Now for another story. (He sings a lusty symphonic theme as he lines up the cows and horses behind the box. The little calf is placed well away on its own. He almost forgets Bull and puts it in place last of all.)

Black Cow and Mother Cow are great enemies and they kick each other. This Bull is a leader, but he's not a good one. Now they all go away. Mother Cow is going to dance with Wild Horse. Now they're loose, doing what they want. Scrambling over each other. They kick the man but he recovers. (Perhaps this man is my husband.) But boy, is he afraid! No one to handle them, and they kick, fight—two bucking horses with men on them. And Flicker dances alone. Dougie, are you writing my thoughts now? The elephant carries the Mother Cow away, and now Flicker. Hey, Mother Cow's going to stand on Flicker. (He sticks them together with plasticine, singing meanwhile 'She likes gin, I like rum, I tell you what, we've lots of fun!' from the song 'Little Brown Jug'.) Now you're writing my thoughts? (that this is a sexual game). Now there's four animals and they all tumble. A horse broke its tail. Oh oh, its Flicker. It's awful to think he got his legs broken. (Sammy thinks sexual ideas are dangerous.) I can't play this any more. It's a great shame. (He starts to trot round the room shouting, 'The cow, the cow, the cow bit the cat's tail off.' He comes back to the table and himself bites the toy cat's tail off with his teeth. The tiger and several of the other wild animals then receive the same treatment.) There that's the end.

Although Sammy would seem to act out an oral castration rather than talk about his penis worries, I feel he has not yet given me sufficient material for interpretation of these anxieties. He is distressed by the sight of the 'castrated' Flicker, an irreparable situation. The oral felicity of the 'Little Brown Jug' song makes me wonder whether this primal scene game is also a reference to real memories concerning Sammy's mother, her drinking problems, and her behaviour towards him at these times. Is Sammy identifying with a bad mother-image who orally incorporates the father's penis?

77

36th Session (Thursday 23.12.54)

S. – I had two dreams last night. One started the minute I was coming up out of the subway to come here. I get in here and you had a triangular-shaped chocolate ice-cream and I ate it with a spoon. You gave me too much and I couldn't finish it all. And sitting on this table was a cow—a regular cow but with fluffy things like feathers or cotton round its head. It was spotted like the Black Cow. Then there was a horse too. I just remember it was there . . . two animals and a cow with fluffy horns. Oh, write the next one down, would you? I keep forgetting that one. I was going under a bridge in a train. You were with me. We were standing at the back of it. Then the train came near the side of a stone bridge. Now let's have our game. That's enough about dreams.

(The games begin as before with kick fights, in which the Black Cow and Mother Cow play the most active roles. Then Flicker is taken out of the box.)

Oh, I'm just so bored of him. Let's set fire to him so we'll know he's not going to be used any more. It's because of his legs all broken. (He burns Flicker's head with a match.) If we could get his head off we'd know he's not a good horse. Flicker is burnt to do him good. He's no good any more. Now all are happy because there are no more dead people or sick ones. It's good that Flicker is burnt. That does some good around this house. Here's a sign of Flicker. He died and that's his statue, a souvenir of Flicker. It must always be kept there. (There ensue some complicated animal fights, with Bull and the two cows.) This Black Cow is a fine coward. There must be a strong master to keep them calmed. (Sammy feels a strong father-person is needed.) And the Black Cow is thought by the people to deliberately kill two people. No master to take care of them. All loose now. The villain (a soldier with a gun) sticks Black Cow with his sword in the back. There now. In the stomach and in the side. Old Black Cow he's wounded and off he goes to the cows' hospital. This horse doctor says 'Never, never do that again.' Black Cow is too dumb to be sorry he killed the calf. He's back home. Too much for a big day.

37th Session (Friday 24.12.54)

Today on opening the box of toys Sammy finds to his immense shock a child's drawing in there. I am equally surprised, since no one

78

uses these toys but Sammy, who is by far my smallest patient. (I learn later that one of my own children had been looking at the toys the night before, and no doubt for good reasons of her own, had left this memento.)

S. – Ha! Now what is that? What — is — it!! Who's been in my box? (He looks at me accusingly.)

J. M. – (A bit feebly.) Well, what does it look like?

S. – It's another boy's drawing. What was he doing here? Did he touch the Black Cow? He'd better not touch the Black Cow!

J. M. – I think you are jealous of other children who might spend time with me here.

S. – Now, I gotta be careful and throw all the wild animals back into the box.

J. M. – I think it's because you're hurt and angry at me, and so you're taking care not to hurt me.

S. – Well, we'll just go on with our game. (I mention this small interlude because it probably has some effect on the jealousy theme which soon develops in the game.)

All the animals are eating and the Bull doesn't care for Mother Cow. Black Cow is too busy eating to care about the Bull. Bull kicks Mother Cow. Black Cow kicks Bull. Oh, that Mother Cow, the bad, the very bad cow. She's not so nice. The Bull and her are about the same. They're to fight now because it's the fall . . . the fighting season to see who will be head of the land. Everyone hopes that Wild Horse will win. All the others gather round to watch. Mother Cow is smart, and knows many things to tell her calf, even if it was dead. And she told Bull it was the fighting season for them. There goes Wild Horse and Black Cow. He lost, Black Cow did, and he's gone away. He was too ashamed to show his look. (Sammy makes sexual confusions perhaps to protect himself against anxious thoughts.) Wild Horse is king of the land. A hurricane comes. The tallest and strongest trees get blown down. Now Black Cow and Bull will fight. (Black Cow has again become 'she' and the fight that follows is fiercely dramatic, much the most explosive to date and so rapidly announced that I can note very little of it. Whenever I stop writing down his words, Sammy immediately shouts at me to continue. I must not remain unoccupied!) Black Cow badly hurts Bull, and he creeps up on her while she's at her hay. Bull is shivering with

fright. He jumps, attacks lots and lots of times. (Interpret—dangerous male-female sexual exchange.) Black Cow is unconscious and
fainted, and everyone goes away from her. Her back legs are paralysed all over so she can't move, and the animals wouldn't give her a
drink for six months. (Interpret later, that people like me who do
things with other people, children, husband, besides Sammy, would
be better off paralysed so they couldn't move about and do harm.) A
day has passed and Bull and Black Cow are nervous. Bull is more
nervous though, because that Black Cow is really vicious. Black Cow
is missing all the fun as her punishment, and she's getting high fevers
up to 102. Such bad temper and it's had a rough life. And the man
has to give him a shot right in its shoulder. Penicillin shot, tetanus
shot, diphtheria shot and smallpox vaccination. Starts to move his
back legs. In a day his fever will be over. Bull is ready to jump and
paralyse it again if it gives any trouble. No one blames Bull. Black
Cow staggers around, he's been unconscious for six years and doesn't
remember all this.

The end of the game is confused. Different people try to ride the
Black Cow and fall off. Instead of having the story read back Sammy
asks if I will just write an ending to it, and put down 'a good ending . . . the best of all.' Out in front of the waiting-room, Sammy
begins a pantomime where he is falling and staggering around.

J. M. – Who are you now?
   S. – I'm the Black Cow!!

> Sammy struggles today with feelings of jealousy and
> aggression. Black Cow-Dougie is to be kept in order by Bull-
> Father, but she continues to be dangerous. Perhaps Sammy
> restores me at the end when he identifies with Black Cow.
> This way we are both protected against his destructive
> feelings.

38th Session (Saturday 25.12.54)

(This was Christmas Day. Although I was taking a week off,
Sammy's mother begged me to continue seeing Sammy if possible,
because without school or analytic sessions it would be hell and
torture for all the household. Since I was staying in Paris I agreed to
see him through the holiday. Sammy had talked a lot of the Christmas

present he wanted to give me, and asked many questions about what I intended to give him. He said he would like 'candles and something else too'. In spite of anticipating catastrophic reactions to any presents I might give him, I felt his frustration at receiving nothing would be even worse. I bought him a very large coloured candle and a box of sweets.)

S.–Ah, today it's our Christmas party. (He notices some small candles which I have placed around the chimney, ready for lighting.) Oh, how gorgeous! I know, let's get all the animals out too. There's going to be a big fire, but we'll save it till the last minute. Now here's the matches all ready. You sit back and write my thoughts. You know my thoughts better about the fire than some of the other things. Now shall I light it? No, wait a bit. It's hard to think. Oh I just can't do it. Oh, I have to do it! I'm going to force myself to do it! The fire is there just for us. The cows are going to start their game just like any other day. Black Cow is not kicking because of her last experience. He'll try to do it, and just see what happens! (The animals are now led up in a group to watch the lighting of candles and the 'fire'. Sammy picks up Black Cow and says, 'This cow is being burnt', and he starts to look quite anxious. He turns round to me and shouts).

    S.–Go on writing! You've been watching too long. Go on, I'm
        dictating. I'm your dictator! Will you write *please*!
J. M.–What do you want me to write?
    S.–That I'm playing with fire, and what I'm doing and what I'm
        thinking.

(I write that Sammy gets very excited when there is a fire, and he thinks always that he is doing something naughty. That makes him cross with me. He wants to burn Dougie-Black Cow because of all the bad feelings he has given her.)

    S.—All the animals line up and gather round for a fine Christmas
        time. All the animals now go back into the box. Except this
        one. (He picks up the Black Cow and passes her through the
        candle flame and then she too is laid down. He says goodbye
        to all the animals before leaving.)

In accordance with Sammy's instructions I opened his Christmas gift after he left. He had chosen a bottle of perfume shaped like a heart called 'Coeur de Joie'.

39th Session (Monday 27.12.54)

S. – Did you like my present?

J. M. – Yes. Thank you very much.

S. – No thanks for yours! I don't like *any* sweets. And the candle was no good because it overflowed. My mother was pretty mad with you for giving me things I don't like!

J. M. – I think any presents I give you would be frightening and disappointing to you Sammy.

S. – Now that's enough! Let's get on to the games. These cows — I have better ones at home. Just give me a jar of water. That'd be a nice present!

J. M. – Sammy, I think you would find it dangerous to like anything that I give you. You would like lots of things but at the same time you are frightened of getting them.

S. – Well, my mother thinks you give me things I don't like.

J. M. – It's easier for you to love Mummy and to hate me.

S. – I wish you wouldn't talk so much.

He now begins his game to a Beethoven theme and lines up the animals. Bull and Black Cow begin to kick each other but he arrests their movement, and suddenly begins to place them around in an apparently aimless formation.

S. – Did you see what I just did?

J. M. – Yes, but I don't understand what is happening.

S. – Look. (He takes a pencil and draws around the group of cows. It makes a figure 8. He has two other groups which I am to guess, and which turn out to be 7 and 10.) It was just to make a more interesting show. (Then follows a game in which the animals simply come out and go back into the box — even the wild ones). There, that story was well written.

J. M. – Perhaps you liked those two games because nothing really happened, and nobody got angry.

S. – Oh, I'm very pleased with this game. Now a story about Wild Horse. A brand new fresh thoroughbred, and people are getting him on to a ship.

On the boat there is a little boy called Alex. Alex feeds Wild Horse who turns round motionlessly. He's getting nervous and kicks his stable and is very wild. There's a fire and the boat starts to sink. Night time. Wild Horse kicks to the shore. Alex is with him. Now he's going to train him to be a real tame horse. He kicks and rears and jumps off. (The horse is taken from the scene.) Alex cries, 'Oh, I lost the Wild Horse. I lost him.' He whistles but nothing came. One day he finds him drinking. This horse begins to get tame. Alex rides bareback. 'No my boy, I'm not going to fall off you! You better be calm.' Wild Horse thought, 'Well, no point in rearing up. I'd better be good.' Then their house starts to burn. Alex throws pails of water on it, and then rides his horse away. Wild Horse kills another horse. It's the fighting season. Alex bandages him all up, and asks his parents if he can keep him because he's tamer now. (Sammy is being kinder to his instinctual 'wild' self.) The farmer puts it with the other horses. They have a race and another horse strikes him and makes his foot bleed but he wins. Now all go back for a happy time.

J. M. – Well that's all the time we have now.

S. – No. No! (He jumps around screaming madly that he will not leave. He seizes the papers saying his mother will read the story back if I don't and starts hitting me wildly.)

J. M. – You know Sammy I think you're a bit like the little Wild Horse. You want to be tame but you don't want to lose your wild feeling either.

S. – (Suddenly calm.) Ah yes, I understand this horse very well.

Sammy says goodbye and goes off smiling.

As I had expected the exchange of Christmas gifts made Sammy anxious. Besides no material gift could dispel his deep feeling of lack and deprivation. Everything he asks for is so mixed with frightening aggressive feelings that he can't allow himself any fulfilment. His mother once told me that he had asked last Christmas for 'an ideal Christmas tree', that is one which would touch the ceiling. On Christmas day he discovered such a tree in their dining-room, hung with little gifts he and his mother had bought together. He was forced to denigrate the tree, saying it was too big, and spent the day with an insignificant toy tree given by a neighbour.

40th Session (Tuesday 28.12.54)

I read yesterday's story back, with interpretations touching Sammy's identification with Wild Horse, and also with the little boy who wants to tame Wild Horse, and save him from dangers like fire, that is, exciting and forbidden games. Sammy listens with the calm reserved only for listening to his stories with 'thoughts' included. At no other time is he really tranquil for more than two seconds. He finds a new horse and a new cow which I had promised him.

S. – Oh new ones! Now for a new story!

These new animals are to be animals that don't kick. Unless anyone comes too close to them, that is. The Black Cow kicks the New Horse who kicks back. Black Cow is kicked over. Nobody minds! New Cow kicks Bull. It kicks for the very first time. Bull is trying to get the Black Cow on its feet because it has fainted. New Horse is friends with people who don't bother it all the time. (Sammy feels a bit bothered by me all the time. Perhaps he has to be a bit wild here to protect himself, and so as not to get too bothered.) New Horse says, 'That Bull was driving me mad'. Little Calf isn't here. This story is like real life. When people die they don't come to life again. The Black Cow hasn't calmed down since the early days. How I remember those days when I used to get bored! (He now advances all the animals on to the paper I am writing his story on.) Black Cow tramples on everyone. (He suddenly starts to laugh very loudly.) Keep on writing. Just write round the animals whatever they do. The trees are shining in the sky. Look at New Horse! (He giggles again, quite shrilly.) Black Cow and the others all drop out to find out what's the matter. You know what's wrong? (He goes off again into peals of giggles.) It's getting worse and worse. Well, each one finds out. It doesn't seem so good. Not at all! The animals won't tell. They can tell the man. The man's going to tell everyone in the village what is wrong with New Horse. All the people gather round to hear. (Sammy is once more convulsed with laughter.) Every soul on earth has found out what's the trouble with New Horse. They tease him for the thing he did. Dougie, you know what it is? You're sure you don't know? Promise? The people all tell themselves they won't say it out loud. The prince knows it's not serious, but it's something that shouldn't be done. (He explodes with laughter, and rolls round in his chair.) I . . . I can't say it. I want to, but I can't. I don't like to.

J. M. – Are you scared of what I might think?

S. – Yes. Perhaps you mightn't appreciate it.

Oh man, oh man, I can't tell! Now I'm going to tell. Oh I can't! I might get put in jail if I tell. Oh, oh, oh my landlord! Even the Calf in heaven is watching. Well now, I'll find out, if this old prince gets out of the way. (The 'prince' is driven off the table with force.) New Horse backs away. The people find it's getting so horrid. They all tease it. The horse is really ashamed but he keeps on *doing* it. It's a real trouble. That's the trouble. It's getting worse, like a hurricane. (Sammy turns to me.) Oh, but you can't know in which way I mean 'hurricane' . . . oh, I can't, I can't. I wish I could tell you. Are you writing all my thoughts? If I tell you, you'll know all my thoughts. Oh, I should only tell my parents a thing like that, but I can't ever. Since you're a psychoanalyst I can tell you. (He takes a deep breath, but looks rather agitated.) This horse is so ashamed he can't bear it . . . oh oh oh . . . (Sammy rolls from his chair on to the floor as though in mortal agony, holding his stomach with his hands.) Now, I must. Oh, help. Now the change is coming in this story. He gallops. It gets worse and worse. (Sammy rolls over on the floor groaning and moaning and makes little masturbatory movements.) Oh man, oh ladies! What is going to happen if I tell?

J. M. – Sammy, what do you think might happen?

 S. – I might get put in jail. You might send me away to a German camp where they do brutal things to you. Now. Oooooh! (He screws himself up to tell his secret.)

Do you know . . . oh . . . this horse—keep on writing! (He laughs and then begins to babble, but again makes an effort to talk to me.) Oh man, I can't. You must know what it is! I wish I could get this thought out of my head. It's nothing. Just something to make the world spin with a lot of talk. I'll cry if I go home without telling you. Oh, it's so difficult. (He struggles for several minutes more with his thought. Time is up, but he seems so overwrought that I let him continue talking.) Write my thoughts at the same time while I tell. Everybody found out and knew. Now they're going to give this horse a slap, kick and punish. It won't do this awful thing ever again. It's going to cry and cry and cry. And this horse . . . (again he starts off several times to tell me). This horse was walking in the street one day. He heard something . . . a farty noise . . . and he had diarrhoea. He went fart-fart in his tail. (He repeats this 5 or 6 times.) Lots of diarrhœa-ish and things like that. It got so sick in the head. It went into everyone's face till the horse was empty of all things. All it's bad

85

feelings went out. And you are going to tell me that all mine went out too. (His voice is much calmer now, but he is still very worked up.) People died from its fart-fart getting into their insides. It's terrible fart-fart! One by one they all died because the dishorrœa-ish went all over. He went until he made it all over everyone. Then never never again. (Sammy looks anxiously up at me.)

J. M. – We'll see tomorrow why it was so difficult to tell.
    S. – It's a very bad thing. It made such dishorrœa-ish it is terrible. It's going to be killed soon! Bad, bad, bad, bad. It won't ever do it again.

Thursday 30.12.54

At the time of Sammy's session Mrs Y phones to say that Sammy has had a high fever ever since his session on Tuesday. The doctor does not know what caused it, but he is now almost back to normal and can go out tomorrow if he has no temperature. Sammy then comes on the phone and asks me many times why he fell ill and what I thought about our last session. I reassure him over the fart-fart stories and tell him there is no need for him to feel poisoned by them and to have fevers. I also say that maybe he thinks I made him ill since I allow him to talk about these things. 'O.K. Dougie I guess I can come back tomorrow.'

> Sammy's story about the galloping horse and his gestures all indicated intense masturbatory excitement, but he expresses his excitement in a richly intricate *anal* fantasy. It is, of course, the sadistic rather than the erotic dimension which comes to the fore in the story. Sammy feels that his 'bad' feelings (equated with dangerous faeces) will kill everybody including the people he loves. This is described in Sammy's tale as an anal loss. 'Horse is empty of all things. All his bad feelings went out.' 'Any desire for close contact with others will kill and will be punished by death' would seem to be an underlying theme.

41st Session (Friday 31.12.54)

Sammy seems undecided about beginning a game. Opens the box, closes it again.

S. – No! This story will not have any music. Oh, it's a great shame to come here. I didn't want to come here.

J. M. – Perhaps you were worried about the fart-fart and the diahorrœa stories.

S. – Where's New Horse. (He places it in the centre of the table and all the animals around it in the circle. He ponders this scene a while then removes the horse and puts it on the floor.)

All the animals are taking a nice walk. (He reaches down and again adds the horse to the group of animals. Then picks up the new cow and examines it minutely, smiling to himself all the while. He starts to sing.) A trouble is flying through the air. A trouble, a trouble, is flying, oh my goodness, is flying through the air. No one knows what it is. (He examines with care the tail of the new cow.) A trouble's flying through the air. Everyone's come to find out what the trouble is. Everyone's going round this cow. Now the Scientist comes along. (He looks up at me smiling almost coyly, as he places a farmer with a stick in his hand, next to the cow.) Ah, this New Cow. There's trouble with it! (This he repeats four times.) All the animals gather round this cow's back end. Everyone knows the trouble, (sings air from Norwegian Wedding Day). Oh me, that's another thing to tell you. Oh my darling, if I get put in jail I won't laugh. It's an even worse trouble than the other one had. But this one didn't do it, but it *has*!

J. M. – What has it done?

S. – No, it's not done anything. It *has* it. Speech, speech! Everyone's pushing to see. It's . . . oooooh! (He falls on to the floor writhing as though in pain.) Oh, what can I do. I can't say it! (He peers out from under the table at me, and ducks back in again like a baby playing peep-bo.) Oh me, oh my, that's a real trouble with that cow. (He climbs back on his chair and grabs a pencil making as if to stab the cow with it, but changes his mind and lays the pencil down.) This cow is going away, animal-with-a-trouble! It's running away (he sings very loudly) running, running, it can't run. It's tumbled from the trouble it has. Oh it's going to be hard. It's crying. The cow is crying. Oh darling, it's going to be sad at the end. Oh my men, my me! 'Stop the fart-fart,' they said to the New Horse. The trees are shining in the sky. Then the cow does a . . . oooh men! New Horse goes on with its fart-fart, and now all the people have pinned it in, so it will stay inside him. When he's ready not to go we'll take it off.

But there's this worse trouble with the cow. (The last few movements have been accompanied to Rimsky-Korsakov's Coq d'Or Suite. Knowing that Sammy spends hours listening to his records, I have sometimes asked him why he chooses one theme or another, but he always shakes his head with a little frown, to indicate that this is a private domain. But on this occasion he begins to sing Beethoven's Funeral March, staring at me fixedly all the while.)

J. M. – Why are you singing the Funeral March, Sammy? (Sammy does not reply, but points dramatically to the cow.)

J. M. – You think she'll get killed for this? (Sammy nods vigorously. He switches to singing a theme from the Pastoral Symphony and brings out the New Horse.)

S. – New Horse is now the leader. But that cow (picks it up) — this was a brave cow (again intones the Funeral March).

J. M. – We don't have much more time now. (Sammy remains in the same position staring at the animals, looking very undecided. After some hesitation he puts down the cow.)

S. – I wish I were a different person and wouldn't have all these troubles. (With a sudden change of tone and a little gesture as though to throw all the 'troubles' on to me.) Oh, it's more a trouble about you than it is about me! You don't care about me. That's what!! I never heard of such a thing. A psychoanalyst caring about her own self and not about other people! My other psychoanalyst loved me more than all the rest. She thought I had interesting little ways. (He menaces me with his fists.)

J. M. – You're afraid I don't love you because of your thoughts. These thoughts are hard to say, and that makes you angry with me. You think Dr G was nicer. She didn't make you talk about all these frightening ideas.

S. – The trouble is ... oh ... (His voice almost disappears, and he makes a few little squeaky sounds, while he gestures helplessly.)

J. M. – You can tell it tomorrow if you like.

S. – (Jumping up from his chair and clutching me with both hands.) Stay, stay, you must listen. I can't go on like this! Keep on writing!! (He seems midway between play-acting and panic so I sit down again, and start to write.)

This great big fat chubby young cow, pretty as she is . . did the great trouble, which is — oh merde! — which is that this cow has a big fat swollen udder, and the second thing is that this cow has a bleeding behind. And its bladder doesn't feel too well, and its behind is very hot, and this cow's not feeling too well. It's a bad cow! And the important thing it did . . . oh this is even a worse trouble . . . (to me: 'write, write!') it did so vomit all over the grass and people and babies and every little thing. Since it vomited it got sicker and sicker and the name of its bad fever is tetanus. It's shaking all over. Mouth closed, got a hot tongue and a big fat behind with no fart-fart, just a little smell. And it felt sorry. This cow is a good cow. No one knows. Next year on January 3rd, the Wild Horse might have a trouble and before January 16th all the animals might have a trouble. It will be one of my greatest troubles! Everybody might be dead including the horse and the sick cow. It is such a good cow — and a bad one. All the gathering gave it a good kick and medicine, and everything's fine with it. A good cow, the best of all.

J. M. – We will have to stop there for today.

   S. – No! No! I won't go! You must let me stay or I will get sick. Last time I had a fever because of the same reason. I will be ill again the same way if you send me home. (Screaming) Do you want me to get a fever?

J. M. – You will not get a fever, nor any of the sicknesses of the cow or the horse. We will understand all these things together.

Sammy's cow with her swollen udder and bleeding behind contains a damaged and frightening image of femininity, and possibly a reference to the mother's pregnancy. In any case the aggressive oral incorporation fantasies bring about a need for oral ejection. (Did Sammy's mother visibly suffer from morning-sickness when pregnant with the second child?)

42nd Session (Monday 3.1.55)

   S. – Now I must get the right music for the story. Let's see if I can find a magic base. This story is called 'Adventure with Three Troubles in it'.

I know what the troubles are, but they haven't flown through the air yet. Little red flies are shining in the sky. Since it's trouble and

89

excitement we shall play—Grieg! No, that's not right. Bach, the Sonata for Piano and Violin. I will sing the Funeral March only if the story gets too sad. The trouble starts with him and him. (He designates Wild Horse and Fart-Fart Horse.) The troubles are starting to fly through the air. Green grasses are flying, and papers and no one knows. (To me.) I got another fever from not telling all my troubles! The trouble is now with this Wild Horse. Have a good look at him! (He is held near my face for inspection.) Him and Fart-Horse are going to fight. This bad Fart-Horse will be called after his troubles. (The horse is tapped solemnly and Sammy chants the Funeral March over him.) Can you see what's wrong with Fart-Fart Horse? He had the pin in his behind, but now it comes out, and all the air comes too. Finally they put a piece of wood across the behind of his highness. Now it's the fighting season for who's going to be king of the land. Wild Horse wins, but oh, his trouble is showing! (Chants the Funeral March.) The leaves are flying through the air. Oh oh my met! (Sammy falls on the ground writhing and sighing, and mock sobbing.) Oh, the animals smell it! The horse is warm on its back. Oh it's a good fine trouble. Will you please close your eyes while I prepare the trouble of the Wild Horse? (He sticks plasticine on its tail.) It's backing away so people won't bother it. (Sings Grieg lustily.) The trouble is . . . oooooh . . . it's giving me a pain in my heart. It's going to kill my heart. Oh darling, I don't know. I thought I could. Oh the trouble is . . . well . . . oh, if I turn the horse around ooooooooh (he simulates noisy crying). Oh, it's giving me pains all over. It's going to be hard and painful. I must tell it! I must! This horse . . . it's too difficult . . . I wish I could tell you . . . but I can't. I can. I must! (Noisy tearless sobbing.) Oh darling . . . it's . . . oh darling this horse . . . if I don't tell . . . it's diarrhœa-ish . . . all its BMs (Sammy's childhood word for bowel movement) . . . but that's not the trouble . . . the worst is when it makes big swollen intestines like a bellyful of soup. Look at it! It's going to die!! It's behind is the biggest hindest hurting behind. It feels like it's sticking pins and needles in its behind. Hurting bad. Oh don't cry! Don't! There's a little gas from it and diarrhœa-ish dripping all over. He's stepped and rolled over it and got it on his belly. Crying because it fell over. Laughing, crying and screaming. Didn't know what it was doing. Everyone was afraid of this horse and its tail. And its mouth full of diarrhœa. It's so sick it doesn't know what. It can make double farts of love and sadness, this horse. And its biggest trouble is the hot air coming out of its mouth. This horse is a bad horse. All the trouble is over! (Sammy then writes on the page himself: It is a good horse and a bad horse.)

Sammy's eyes are full of anxiety at the end of the session, but as we read his story back he becomes calmer. I try to show him how he uses a confusion between bottoms and mouths to protect himself from 'flying apart'.

> I think his excitingly explosive anal-erotic fantasies arouse fears of losing his body-identity. His 'oh darling—this horse—all its BMs' suggests that Sammy could be dramatising a mother who is frightened by her baby's anality. I think Sammy regards my interpretations also, as frightening 'hot air'.

43rd Session (Tuesday 4.1.55)

    S.–Hey, are you eating something? You haven't much lipstick on. Go and put it on!

J. M.–Why do you ask me that?

    S.–Because . . . because . . . (He menaces me with his fists.) I want you to, see? You better do it, or else (he approaches seemingly prepared to kick me) . . . and your hair too. It looks messy. You look awful. Go and do these things or else . . . (His voice rises to a scream, and then he subsides into his chair.) Well, I won't tell you any stories today. I'll read instead.

J. M.–It seems to me that you would like to avoid the ideas in the stories like the hot air that came out of Fart-Fart Horse's mouth.

    S.–I want to talk to a nice clean psychoanalyst, who has lots of lipstick on.

J. M.–Perhaps you think the story ideas aren't 'clean' because they're about BMs? I listen to the stories with you so maybe you think I'm not clean either.

    S.–(As though struck by a sudden inspiration.) Have I been forgetting the bulls? Now where's that Bull. (He extracts Bull and Black Cow.) We must make sure we have all the animals.

There are eleven of them. Now for the music . . . I know . . . Peer Gynt.

Mother Cow and Bull aren't getting along well these days. It's because Mother Cow wants to rub its horns against the back of Fart-Fart Cow (the New Cow of session 41) because she's got such a nice sort of bottom. Her horns are always itching these days. He rolls over and over in the grass. Mosquitoes and fleas are bothering him. He's itching all over. (The animals are placed in a circle.) By the way, Black Cow is acting better these days. Here's Bull cantering, in a dancing sort of way. Oh the little green leaves are flying in the sky. (He sings this phrase over many times, then switches abruptly to the Funeral March, looking fixedly at me again. He turns his attention to Bull, tapping it slowly to indicate that the 'troubles' for today reside in him.) The animals circle round Bull. A horse advances and whinnies around Bull's behind, then drops back into place. A fierce fight between Mr Bull and Mother-Cow. Ah ha! Mrs Young Cow isn't too pleased. She wants New Horse's behind all to herself. She's jealous of the other horse who is interested in New Horse's behind. Whoever wins the fight can have this horse's behind and keep it for a pet. The horse's behind is here, waiting like that, it's facing them. Now Bull and Mother-Cow start their great angry fight. The winner gets the horse's behind. And friends can have it also, and can lick and rub their horns against it. One of Bull's kicks gets into the Cow's stomach. It's bleeding. But strong and gay as ever, and very angry. It's hard for Bull to keep up because it has a trouble too. Cow wins!! She rubs her sore feet on his behind. She's a good rubber. (Sammy then mimes the cow rubbing its nose around the bull's behind, but does not verbalise this. I announce that this is the end of the session and Sammy begins to put up his usual resistance to leaving, and a lot of pantomime about telling the 'Trouble'. There is more play-acting than panic now, but he is nevertheless tense and anxious.) This time the Bull's trouble . . . oh darling it's going to be difficult . . . etc. Oh, it's giving me a pain in my liver! Just see if you can tell what it is. It's got to do with his intestines. Mother-Cow laughs and mucks about in Bull's behind. Because that's where the trouble is. Bull's awful trouble is that it has a behind all green and the important part where the BMs come out . . . oh . . . it's all purple. And it has a cow fever, called . . . ah . . . Harpuschondriaca. It has a dirty behind. Now write down my thoughts too! Good Bull is such a dirty Bull.

92

But next time he'll be nice. This cow is a bully. She has a trouble too. She'll be so afraid. Bull goes sadly away with his sad thoughts. And this was a very good idea. And everybody goes home. The end!

Sammy makes no more objections to leaving. The detailed expansion of his fantasies seems to have helped him.

The exchange of anal parts and products in today's story tend towards a phallic representation, and are I think, an appeal to the Father (as when Sammy suddenly realises he has forgotten Bull). But thereafter the maternal image once again fills the whole scene. As in the previous session the drama becomes centred on one cow's horns and another cow's behind. The ambiguity of these two maternal images is evident. Sammy plays out a fantasy of the primal scene in which the two protagonists are identified within the phallic mother, the phallic quality being expressed in anal terms.

Under cover of the anal material with which he now feels relatively safe, Sammy can embark on a situation which is more oedipal when he brings into play the Bull and it's rivalry with Horse. In this new triangular relationship the content is clearly pregenital. The anal form of the stories also serves as a narcissistic protection. The 'horse's behind' for which the two animals fight represents in all probability Sammy himself. In the normal course of events the little child invests the faecal part-object demanded of him by his mother with immense significance. In addition to its libidinal significance it represents also a new dimension in his sense of separate identity. Mother wants something from him which he is free to give or withhold. He is an individual who can frustrate or fulfil another's desire. It seems that Sammy was never able to take this important step towards separate identity perhaps feeling that his mother, because of her own unconscious needs would not survive such a separation. This situation is personified in the role of Mother Cow who wins total proprietary rights over the little horse's behind (while Father-Bull is excluded). In fact in the next session Sammy even calls New Horse 'Flicker', the horse with which he previously identified himself. In other words he is the part-object belonging only to Mother and which she won after the primal scene.

93

44th Session (Thursday 6.1.55)

S. – (Pointing to Black Cow.) Oh boy, is this one having trouble!
(She is tapped to the strains of the Funeral March.) Black Cow's
dancing up and down. Black Cow's got a bleeding leg because of its
fighting. Now Mother Cow comes over and sniffs at the behind of
New Horse, because you remember what happened last time. (He
refers to the fact that Mother Cow won the horse's behind.) Now all
the animals run away because a very bad thing happened to all these
trees. They had poison in them. (He taps a round apple tree, singing
the Funeral March upon it. The pantomime about telling the trouble
starts again and is finally announced.) This tree trouble is BMs
which came out of Flicker. (The name of 'Flicker' has now been
conferred upon New Horse which has also been called Fart-Fart
Horse.) Black Cow stamps angrily. (Funeral March.) She doesn't
like having a trouble. Her trouble is entirely different. Oh my
darling . . . oh . . . oh . . . (etc. for some minutes). Oh my appendix
ache! My darling, my appendix . . . when I get fevers all the time . . .
darling darling I might have a heart attack when I get home. Oh
dear I'll get thrown in jail, thrown in the camp fire, caught by
cannibals. Oooh, I'm getting heart attacks, my head has a trouble
it's turning into wood! Keep writing, keep writing! When I see you
writing, I can tell the trouble. This famous trouble is very difficult . . .
(etc., for some further time) Black Cow has two big fat lumps on its
behind because it's got a sickness called Horgen and Highen, tail
aches, and stomach gas that goes up. He's aching all over. He has
arm-ache too because he has swollen diphtheria. (To me.) That's your
head! He's got a big fat swollen leg near its behind. From its behind
white stars and leaves are flying through the air. Black Cow doesn't
know the reason for its terrible thoughts. Its horns hurt. It's all
caused by trouble it had when it was young. This bad trouble, it
won't get it again, because now this nice horse rubbed its behind. No
more fevers now. It's going to be all better soon.

Sammy-Flicker makes poisonous BMs, that is, gives back in
a bad form the good food he incorporated. This will kill all the
others. But Sammy and Dougie are both Black Cow too, they
have troubles with their heads. There is a 'horrible trouble' of
confused relationships but we see at the end that a helpful anal
introjection from a father-image will be healing to Black Cow-

analyst, and more especially to Black Cow-Sammy, 'because this nice horse rubbed its behind'.

45th Session (Friday 7.1.55)

Sammy asks for the story to be read back with his thoughts put in. I give him an interpretation about his fantasies of exchanges between himself and me. His desire to get good things from me and fear of their turning out to be very bad once they are absorbed by him; (the BMs that poison everyone) and his need for helpful strong people against the frightening images of himself or me.

S.–Oh, you forgot to mention the day I hit you on the head with the White King. I was too frightened then to tell you all these stories. (Sings the Funeral March and makes signs over the Wild Horse and the Black Cow.) But today New Cow has troubles. I remember all the troubles she already had (swollen udders). While all the animals are hungry they eat at the trees. New Cow and Mother Cow play together. Oh, he does have a trouble! I know now what it is. There's two troubles, and the second one is a very funny and bad trouble. Keep on writing. Oh darling, I'm getting a lung-ache. You know how it can happen. Lungs can burst!

J. M.–Really?

S.–Oh yes. It's already happened to me. Oh darling, now I'm beginning to get earache because of the trouble. Oooooh. My kidney ache (writhing around as though in great pain). A trouble's flying through the air. Stars are flying in the sky because of this cow's troubles. He's fighting with Flicker, that Warm-Behind horse. He has blank on his blank! Mother Cow is jealous to see New Cow rub its horns on Flicker's behind. Now they are tired of his behind and they want Wild Horse's hole. You know which hole I mean? Well they like to put their heads right in its hole to keep it warm. The horse's hole is waiting for them. And now the two cows will fight for the horse's hole. This trouble-maker New Cow won the fight. So now it will stick its head in the horse's hole. You know what I mean? (Turning to me with a slightly frightened look.) There, in, in. (He mimes this last little scene with loud cries, and moans, jabbing the cow's nose meanwhile all around the behind of the horse. The material suggests so strongly primal scene anxiety and mimicry that I ask Sammy where one might witness games such as these. He falls to the ground groaning.) Oh oh oh. I can't tell. Nobody. Oh darling, the horse didn't like it when the cow licked the hole. (Funeral March.) Now the troubles can be told. If I tell I'll get tied to a tree and crucified. I might start a new religion. If I were famous enough I'd be on God's right side! The trouble is I don't feel like being crucified and put into a coffin!! Oh I might get crucified by those bad people who live in my house. I'll have nails stuck in me! Oh I don't care for it.

J. M. – What is the terrible thing you have done? (I note that this punitive fantasy seems to have been mobilised by my suggestion that Sammy had *watched* the primal scene.)

S. – In the year one, something like that happened. I want the knife stuck in my right side rather than my left. The trouble is (he nurses the cow in his hands, rocking and crooning) very bad, this trouble, very very bad. It's giving me headaches. I might get put on the cross because of this trouble. Well, the less important trouble is that it has a baked behind, on the left side. It hurts very much and is all cold. They put it in the ice-box. It looks bad, but it never had that ever again. And secondly it has cream caramel on its udders. So all the people, judges, kings and queens, and all the bishops come to lick its udders. It even licks its own. A bad trouble because the caramel comes from its belly button. It's dripping all over him. They put chili sauce over it, on its udders and its bottom. Soon it all drips off. After days and days. And the cow drank up its own burnt udders. It was sorry that it did it. They put it in the freezer like jelly. The cow was all better. There were no more troubles.

J. M. – Well we don't have any more time now. (It was already well past the time, and Sammy was aware of this.)

S. – No, no. I want to say more. (He picks up the pencil and tries to write more of the story himself. He is crying. It is time to go and he feels he has not finished. He writes on the bottom of the page: 'And it was playing and things.')

46th Session (Saturday 8.1.55)

Yesterday's story is read back, and Sammy listens with his habitual rapt interest to his productions, and to the 'thoughts' which I introduce. These are mostly linked to the transference, and to the pregenital fears explicit in the stories. I also refer to the primal scene anxieties.

S. – Well, now, today, the Gentle Cow will have troubles. (He picks up a creche toy which is indeed a harmless gentle-looking creature, and not too realistic.)

Gentle Cow kicks and is kicked back by the others. (He brings out the crocodile and taps Mother Cow with it. Becomes suddenly interested in a small lump on the leg of this cow.) Oh dear, she has a lump. I must burn it off. Quick, quick matches! (He tears off into the waiting-room where there is a box. Having burned off the lump he now wants to set fire to the whole cow. I ask him not to do this, and point out that he wants to burn it because it reminds him of all the dangerous mother-things he is frightened about with me.) Well, let's burn lots of the little animals in its place. Let's burn something else. (He is not nearly as urgent and wildly uncontrolled as on other occasions when he has been intent on fire games. His excitement and anger nevertheless mount very quickly. He stamps around and throws everything on the ground, yelling angrily. Finally, he flops into his chair.)

S. – Oh, it's getting rather boring!

J. M. – Mother Cow's 'lump' reminds you she could have a baby and that makes you want to burn all the little animals.

S. – Well, it's time to go home anyway!

47th Session (Monday 10.1.55)

S. – Today's trouble's going to be difficult. It's something I like and I want to have them. But I can't always.

Sammy takes up a pen and writes in his large childish script, with many mis-spellings: 'I want matches. Would you please give me some. I will not be silly with them.' He signs to me not to open my mouth, but to write a reply.

J. M. – (Writes) 'I am sure you will not be silly with them.'

S. – (Writes) 'I want them so I can be happy.'

J. M. – (Writes) 'What do you want to do with them?'

S. – (Writes) 'I want a fire in the fireplace with you and the cows and horses.'

J. M. – (Writes) 'Alright.'

    S. – (Writes) 'I am happy. Are you?'

J. M. – (Writes) 'Yes.'

    S. – (Writes) 'O.K. We will do it. Yes.'

(I note an interpretation about dangers of verbal exchange, and fire excitement, to be given to him when we re-read the session. He still will not tolerate the slightest intervention on my part in any other form, except on the rarest of occasions.)

Sammy makes a paper fire, and the animals are lined up to watch it.

    S. – The animals are saying it's a bit hot outside. All rushing now. Oh darling, darling what can it be? (He holds up Mother Cow for me to see and sings the Funeral March.)

J. M. – She's having some bad trouble? (Sammy nods several times.)

    S. – Wild Horse and New Cow don't know what's going on around here. But oh, oh now I must tell my trouble. (He comes over and licks my face.)

J. M. – Are you the little calf?

    S. – Well, it'll help me to tell the trouble if I do that. (He bends and sucks my cheek.)

J. M. – It seems as if you would like to feed from me, Sammy? Has that got something to do with Mother Cow's trouble perhaps?

    S. – (Singing Funeral March.) This cow's trouble . . . oh, keep on writing . . . oh . . . darling . . . don't stop writing!

J. M. – You think it would be dangerous for me not to be busy writing?

    S. – Well, it's very dangerous if it's not *written down*.

J. M. – What will happen?

    S. – I might be put in jail. Oh darling, no one knows what the trouble is. (He rolls on the floor groaning. Starts several times to talk, but his voice keeps breaking off in a squeak.)

    S. – Its trouble is, its dearest, dearest trouble is that it has a broken tail. But that's the least bad part. The saddest part is . . . oh dear, oh dear, I might get put in prison. An American in a French prison. And with a burnt behind! Its behind is a real burnt behind. If I'm to go to jail, put me in an English jail. Oh darling, everyone's praying and crying for the cow. A burnt behind from a gorgeous fire fire.

J. M. – How did it get burnt?

S. – After all the BMs and fart-fart it sat on the fire. I might get a
burnt behind. Write write, don't stop. It will help my troubles
end. This cow had diarrhœa-ish in its pants, but now everything's going to be better.

I think Sammy had to become the Little Calf today in order to get
close to me in a safe way and keep the troubling primal scene
fantasies of the last few sessions under control. There are more confused zonal images again today. No doubt these confusions help
Sammy to deal with his aggressive and eroticised world.

48th Session (Tuesday 11.1.55)

I read back yesterday's story, interspersing interpretations to the
effect that Sammy seems afraid of my mouth, and of his bottom, as if
he were afraid I might bite his bottom or his tail; and that he could
get close to me as the little sad calf. He then asks if we can't have
some new toys. And if not, some matches. I tell him there are no
matches left today, and this time he accepts the fact without any
uncontrollable outbursts.

S. – Well then, we'll see what we can do. All the animals are upset.
They are in a small ring, see. They don't like it and are trying to get
out. A bad man is closing them in. And the trees make a blocation.
The animals were wild and got caught. Oh the poor caged animals.
(This is like Sammy who wants to get close to me, and then finds his
wild feelings frightening. He feels caged and wants to get away.)
Black Cow jumps out, and the watch dog gets her back. (Sammy
starts to sing the Funeral March, then with much snickering, and
apparent diffidence, writes on the back of yesterday's story-notes the
following words): 'Oh man. Shit. God dammit. Damit.'

He then returns to his game, picks up Flicker, and comes over and
strokes my arm with Flicker's nose.

S. – The animals now kill all the people. They're loose. Strong
healthy animals. Warm-Behind Horse does most of the work. They
knock down all the trees in the enclosure. One man is left who has a
gun as all the animals stampede. (Sammy needs to feel that he can
be protected against all his strong feelings, and the things that he
thinks could happen between us. He would like to think of a strong
man to protect him.) The horses say they won't hurt the man if he

doesn't hurt them. They attack one last man, now all are dead. The animals eat hay and go to sleep. (Sammy sings the Funeral March as he hides something under the table. Meanwhile, he has tossed all the 'dead men' into my lap.) Ah, now a snake crawls out while the animals are asleep. (He produces from under the table the snake — the first time it has been used in Sammy's games.) It slides around without doing anything for a while. If it touches anybody they will die. If you see the animals with any vibration it means they are going to die. (Funeral March as the snake touches the donkey.) Flicker attacks the snake, and then licks the donkey all over. Oh, how did it happen? Donkey says he's hurting all over. 'A man must have stuck a knife into me!' Flicker says, 'You'll have to lie down for three weeks. You've had a snake sting.' Donkey says, 'Are you ridiculous?' Flicker says, 'I killed it. He stung you on your behind.' Weeks pass and the donkey gets better. (I tell Sammy that there is no more time now.)

S. – Well there's a trouble to tell. I won't be too long. Oh my stomach-ache. You might break my arms off if I tell. Oh my gland-ache. You can see the blood. I'm getting paralysed. I have a back-ache and a bone ache. Oh lady. Oh men. Oh lady. The trouble is . . . ooooh . . . when they were crowded together, very hardly, they banged their hot behinds together. So it made grey on the white horse. Warm-Behind Horse was killing one of the men, because it sat on him with its hot behind. (Sammy thinks of getting close to his father. He thinks his father has strong powerful contents inside him. Sammy would like to share in his father's strength and then would feel less frightened of women, his mother or me, but he feels this is forbidden.) A bone broke! They won't do that ever again. It's so naughty. (Sammy nevertheless feels that these ideas about his father are pretty dangerous thoughts too.) It's so terrible, what they did, they won't ever do it again. It'll just fly back through the air. The End.

The whole sequence of the drama leading from an oedipal situation, passing through a homosexual identification to a two-person relationship indicates the precariousness of Sammy's oedipal structure. The homosexual imagery is again in terms of an anal recuperation — rather than a structured oedipal situation. The real power is still on the side of the phallic mother-figure. The snake represents as much her power as the expression of frightening wishes towards the father's penis. (In the session my pen, which preserves Sammy's stories, is probably invested with phallic significance too.)

49th Session (Thursday 13.1.55)

For the first time Sammy does not ask for yesterday's 'story and thoughts'. He makes signs as soon as he enters the room that I am not to open my mouth. He writes: 'Do you have any matches today? If you don't, I won't be unhappy about that.' He puts his hand fiercely over my mouth, and makes signs that I am to reply in writing. The following conversation is all written. [In view of the length of this written dialogue, Sammy's idiosyncratic spelling has been corrected for easier reading.]

J. M. – No. There are no matches.
    S. – It does not matter. It is not that exciting any more.
J. M. – It might even be a bit frightening?
    S. – No. NOT AT ALL!!!
J. M. – I wonder why you didn't want to ask for matches?
    S. – Because I know that you don't have any.
J. M. – Did you have another reason for wanting matches?
    S. – Because there is a trouble flying through the air.
J. M. – A trouble with people's mouths? With talking?
    S. – It is about your FAT HEAD.
J. M. – What is wrong with my fat head?
    S. – It has bones.
J. M. – Does yours have bones too?
    S. – NO. NO. NO. It has cotton. Much better than your head.
J. M. – If yours is much better it might mean you have a better body than me. Because you are a boy?
    S. – Oh.
J. M. – Is that part of the trouble?
    S. – No no I cannot say. Ask GOD. He knows. Don't ask me.
J. M. – Don't you know what the trouble is?
    S. – No. For the last time, ask GOD. He knows.
J. M. – Who is GOD?
    S. – Part of me and part of you.
J. M. – So part of me and part of you knows the trouble?

S. – Yes. But the part of me that knows the trouble does not want to tell the rest of me.

J. M. – So you and I will have to work it out together?

S. – Yes. Do you think that part of you knows the trouble because God is part of you?

J. M. – Part of me does know about your trouble.

S. – What is it?

J. M. – Some of it is to do with the fart-fart and the BMs. Part is to do with the hot bottom that might get eaten.

S. – No. It is something else.

J. M. – It might be about other parts of your body too.

S. – I am going to heaven now. Goodbye, goodbye. I am very happy because I will be with God. Ha ha. I am happy. I just died.

J. M. – What made you die?

S. – The TROUBLE.

J. M. – Why didn't you answer my last question?

S. – I cannot answer because I am in heaven with God. I am DEAD.

J. M. – You can't write it?

S. – Maybe. Oh oh. It is hard to tell. I might die from it. But I will not worry. God will help me if you can't.

J. M. – Perhaps you think I will be angry if you tell it?

S. – I can tell the trouble if God will help me.

J. M. – Do you want to tell this trouble today?

S. – Yes, I will try.

J. M. – I will not let you die even if you tell it!

S. – Oh, I will, I know.

J. M. – Perhaps you think your body won't have any more troubles when you are dead?

S. – No because then I cannot think.

J. M. – I'm sorry but there's no more time left today.

S. – Oh never mind. It was a nice day today wasn't it?

J. M. – Yes. See you tomorrow.

S. – I prefer not seeing tomorrow. I prefer to stay here.

J. M. – Sometimes it seems you would like to live here.

S. – You are a damn LADY FATHEAD.

(No word was spoken throughout the session, and Sammy went off in a more relaxed frame of mind than he usually does. It seems that the phallic pen is less dangerous than the mouth-anus.)

50th Session (Friday 14.1.55)

Yesterday's game is read back, underlining Sammy's need to be anxious about my body and its contents; and his flight into death.

S. – Ah, but that's yesterday's trouble—your fat head. It's hard, your head, and mine's soft.

J. M. – You seem concerned about the differences between us.

S. – Well, that's not today's trouble. (He picks up the box. I have added to the toys a pink plastic boy, complete with penis, thinking that it might help Sammy to attach his fantasies more directly, instead of having them constantly displaced onto the animals where they might remain somewhat removed from conscious acceptance of his feelings about himself and his environment.)

Oh, the beautiful pink boy! Ah, ah, I know the trouble for today. (He taps the boy to the theme of the Funeral March.) Here comes Broken Tail, and Fart-Fart Horse, stampeding after the Lost Boy. Oh man! The trouble I might get if I'm thrown into the Red Sea. I wouldn't care about it. Nor the Black Sea either. (He sticks a piece of plasticine on the Pink Boy.) All the animals circle round as he floats through the air on this swell day. (Sammy comes over to me, still holding the Boy in the air and licks my cheek, then sucks it.)

J. M. – You would like to eat me as though you were a little boy?

S. – How do you like it?

J. M. – It makes me think that you wonder if I am going to want to eat you up too.

S. – Ooooh, if I become like the Black Cow I shan't like it.

J. M. – You remember, Black Cow was me. Perhaps you think that I will damage you, and then you'd get to be like me. Like a girl. Or you might even disappear and turn into me.

S. – Shut up! (He returns to his game, squeaking and squealing as he holds the Boy up in the air.) Oh, oh, I might get shut in a mouse ranger!

J. M. – What's a mouse-ranger?

S. – Your knuckle-head! Now I want to guess at today's trouble. Oh it's so difficult! Oh darling, oh, oh! (He waves his arms about as though conducting music, singing all the while, then falls on the ground.) Keep writing.

The lion is on the ground. Look! He has a bleeding trouble-mouth. (He is actually holding the *calf* in his hands, no doubt because it is associated with the oral-sadistic images, and feeding dramas.) Oh this trouble it'll give me an appendix and lockjaw, and diphtheria and nose-aches. Or it'll break like happened once really to someone when he was playing with some other boys. Well this boy's trouble—he's got BMs all over his behind and he fell against the cow and it went on her too and he has BMs on his penis now. Like your knuckle-head. But you don't have a penis. You have breasts. I don't want any of those! So this boy wiped his BMs all over the cow and all over his penis. And he cried and screamed because of the BMs all over him. His mother will slap him. Look he's crying now.

51st Session (Saturday 15.1.55)

S.–Read out yesterday's troubles, Dougie, and don't forget my thoughts.

I point out his concern over sexual differences, and say my 'stupid knuckle-head' probably means I have a penis missing. Then I suggest that he is also rather envious of my breasts too, and maybe this situation worries him.

S.–Would you read out again the bit about the breasts. (I do this.) Now read it once more. (I read it again without comment.) Oh I'm glad I don't have breasts!

J. M.–Why is that?

S.–Oh darling . . . because then you might bite off my—(He stops short and points to his penis. He then picks up a pencil, taps my chest and sings the Funeral March.)

J. M.–Is that today's trouble? If I have no penis I might take yours?

S.–Yes. (He jumps towards me and attempts to put his hand down the neck of my jersey. I take hold of his hands and tell him I will not permit him to do that, but that we can talk about it as much as he wants. He tries to suck my jersey but when I again say that these things are to be discussed and not played out, he finally sits down.) Oh oh oh! I might get breasts. That's a real trouble! They might break my behind off. But I have a penis. It's more useful than your breasts! Your breasts are no use—unless you have a baby. I don't want breasts. Oh my penis, I don't want breasts!! Oh I wish I didn't have breasts! (He talks along these lines for some minutes, in a squeaky bizarre voice, in which breasts and penises are equated and confused. He then sits up straight and continues in a more normal tone of voice.) Your breasts might pop! They might bite me.

J. M. – Perhaps you mean you might want to bite them?

S. – No no. But one of the troubles is about your breasts. I'm so frightened. But I'm sure glad I don't have breasts. (He picks up the animals and makes a circle around the Boy. He extracts the giraffe which has a broken leg, and pitches him far away.) We don't want him around.

J. M. – He makes you afraid of damage to your own body, of your penis getting hurt?

S. – Yes! But it's much worse about your breasts. They're not like my mother's. Something bad might come out of them. Am I glad I don't have bosoms! You have breasts and a *hole*. And I only have a penis. (He leads out the crocodile, and taps Gentle Cow with it, singing the Funeral March.) Oh men! Two troubles. Crocodile and breasts! (Picks up Flicker and with loud anal noises backs him towards Bull.) Flicker's going fart-fart all over Bull. (Sammy darts towards me and pushes a ball of plasticine into my jersey.)

J. M. – You're being like Flicker. Wanting to put a sort of BMs-penis into me.

S. – I want to play chess.

J. M. – I think you want your father to protect you here. So I won't be a kind of dangerous mother, you want to make me into a strong father you can play chess with instead.

S. – All my friends play chess. I have lots and lots of boy friends. I wish I didn't have to come here—you with your big fat bosoms! The troubles with the animals are all finished now. But not with you! You have many troubles!!

In spite of his extreme agitation Sammy allowed me to talk directly today without having to write everything down first.

The breast is the important part-object in Sammy's present transference relationship and he reveals constantly his oral fantasy of a breast-penis equation and defences against his desire to have breasts. After reassuring himself that his penis, though menaced, is intact, he attacks the analyst's breasts, saying he fears an anal attack from them. Then shortly after he projects an oral-anal sadistic fantasy when he says 'your breasts might pop'. As we have already seen in the games these are also elements in Sammy's primal scene fantasies, as though father and mother put penis and breast into each other's anuses. Sammy's attempt to put the ball of plasticine into my jersey has several determinants:

(a) a tentative erotic approach arousing sufficient guilt to include an element of self punishment;

(b) preliminary gift of a symbolic penis intended to assuage the angry breasts;

(c) restoration of the incorporated part-object on an oral sadistic level—perhaps an attempt to restore the mother's breast in face of an aggressive paranoid fantasy.

In any case Sammy accepts the interpretation of the protective aspect of the chess game and of his 'boy friends'. But the breasts remain dangerous and still to be dealt with.

52nd Session (Monday 17.1.55)

Stimulated by the imminent inundation of Paris by the Seine, Sammy begins his session in high excitement. He hopes Paris will soon be flooded. He almost forgot to ask that yesterday's story be read back!

S. – But there's something more frightening. My mother wants me to take riding lessons. But I'm not getting on any horse. Oh no I'd rather keep my insides right. Gosh I could break a bone! (castration anxiety is again linked to fears of disintegration).

J. M. – Perhaps you're still thinking your penis is in danger if you do things you like.

S. – Yes I am, but I still won't ride. You see this horse didn't understand—he wasn't a psychoanalyst! Now what shall we play today? Ah yes, these four animals have caught very important diseases. (He picks up the four broken toys, puts them together and chants the Funeral March over them.) Now don't stop writing, you, or I'll do something.

106

Bull has a broken hind leg, Brown Cow has a bad foot, Flicker a worse foot and Wild Horse a burnt nose. They will all be taken care of by the Boy. (I note 'thought' to give Sammy later, that he now feels that even if the animals are damaged they can be healed.) Boy is calling the animals one by one into the operating room. Start with the two sickest. The other two can bear it. Now Boy takes Bull very gently by the horns. Bull is nervous but Boy pats him on the back. (Sammy looks up with a smile and in a polite little voice he has never used before asks, 'Could I have a few sheets of paper please? Two more if you're sure you have enough. Thank you, Dougie.') Now I'm going to draw our hospital. Every room the same, radiator, haystack, manger, toilet. Exits here . . . (He plays for about ten minutes demonstrating a quietness and control I have never seen in him before.) Now we must fix up Bull. Open your mouth, stand still Bull! Bull kicks and Boy slaps but it's just because Bull is getting pain. Boy takes the stuff out of his throat. Ah, a bit of diphtheria, I could tell anyone. Just a bit of a throat. Will soon get better. Bull feels it too. Now he can stand up. Now he looks almost as good as ever. (Sammy is reassured about castration fears. He prefers this to the terror of the disintegrating 'insides'; and on the positive side he feels such damage can be healed. He refers to 'our' hospital and seems to identify with me in this healing prospect.)

53rd Session (Tuesday 18.1.55)

  S. – Could I have a pencil and paper please? There's something that's too hard to tell. I couldn't stay in school this morning (group of three children who have private lessons together) because I was . . . oh dear . . . how will I say it? No! I must try to write it. (He writes: 'I could not stay in school because I was a bit ill', then makes a sign to me to write something.)

J. M. – (Writing) What was your illness?

  S. – (Writing) Nothing. Jest bit tieyard.

J. M. – (Writing) Why is it so hard to tell?

  S. – (Writing) No more cweschins please. (He indicates that we may now talk.)

J. M. – What is frightening about the word 'ill'?

  S. – You might send me to hospital! Now let's get on with our game.

Oh boy! There's trouble coming. But not a hard one. It will scare the animals and the Pink Boy. (He hums the Funeral March and draws an indeterminate shape on a piece of paper, which he subsequently places in the middle of the table.) The animals are stampeding away from this great annoyance. Oh darling! You know what it is? It's not fart-fart. I can certainly tell you that. Ooooh! Everyone's scared. It's so hot. But it's an easy trouble by the way. (Funeral March.) It's so hot. It's a fire, but that's not all. If you go far far down . . . oooh! I won't tell you till the last minute. And there's another trouble too, with the Donkey. And another too. (He points to my breasts.) If I tell the first trouble nothing will happen to me. It's not too bad to tell because it's usual. But the Donkey's trouble will make something happen to me. Because it's an animal, it's unusual. And it can only be told when time's up.

J. M. – Perhaps that's a way of not leaving any more time to discuss the donkey's trouble?

S. – But we're only talking about this first trouble. It's helping my illness. If I have an illness.

J. M. – What about this illness of yours.

S. – Your knucklehead! The Funeral March will now be sung and the trouble told. It's —Mt. Vesuvius! Erupting by the way. Now for a fight between Black Bull and New Cow. They want to see who'll be king. (Sammy is crooning and sounds as though he is crying, then he starts to laugh.)

J. M. – That's all for today.

S. – Alright! The donkey's trouble is that he has a crack in his behind, in his warm behind, and that another animal with a warm tongue gave a lick to the BMs that came out of it.

As he goes out of the door, Sammy insists that I write down that the boy forgave the cow (he corrects it to donkey) for everything it had done. (Sammy's slip of the tongue reveals that he forgives the mother-image for the role he attributes to her in his anal-erotic fantasy; the latter is almost certainly associated with anal masturbation.)

54th Session (Thursday 20.1.55)

Sammy arrives earlier than usual today, meets my own children coming out of the front door, and watches them run down the stairs.

S. – Who are those people? Are they patients? Have you got children of your own? What are they doing here? Etc. . . .

I tell him that there is no reason why he shouldn't be curious about other people he sees at my place, but that as he comes here for his own problems it's better that we concentrate on those. He accepts this frustration fairly well, and then begins a long, very rational discussion on psychoanalysis and his reasons for coming. For once he does not ask me to write down what he says and sits quietly in his chair throughout the session.

S. – You know Dougie, I wish I didn't have any troubles. I want to be like other people. Would you make a list of my troubles for me?
J. M. – What do you think your troubles are?
S. – Well my big trouble is I'm afraid of getting ill inside. And I'm afraid of dying. Then I have a big worry that when I grow up, I'll be very very sad, and not at all like other people. That's a trouble too, because when I grow up I'll have to go to war. I don't want to. Why do people have war?

This conversation on war lasted till the end of the session. He talked about his father's having been in the war, and made various surmises about countries likely to precipitate a war. The whole discussion had a semblance of reality such as he has never evinced before. At no point did his fantasy world disrupt the expression of his ideas. At the end of the session, he takes up the opening theme, and says that it will be nice when his analysis is finished, and he can ask questions about those children he saw today.

55th Session (Friday 21.1.55)

S. – You seem different today.
J. M. – Perhaps you feel differently towards me today.
S. – Oh no, not me! For my part I'm just living away. Just living. I'm sorry you seem that way, but it's not my fault.
J. M. – Maybe you want me to have the troubles for a while?
S. – No no not at all. Oh no. It's just your tough luck. I'm not going to be *your* doctor! I'm too busy worrying about my own parts and troubles. (He picks up the box of toys, humming a theme from the Pastoral Symphony then switches abruptly to

Grieg's Norwegian Wedding Day.) Dougie, you must write it down!

Oh ho this new bull is young and dangerous and kicks everyone who gets near. A very very wild bull. And nervous. When they're young they're really good and nervous. Young Bull's a good healthy one. The old one's going to die soon and Young Bull will be chief. The trouble is, he gets so mad and ferocious he rushes into people and knocks their wits out. Now Young Bull fights with Warm-Behind Horse. Funeral March! We haven't seen Young Bull kick yet. But Big Bull likes to keep people from trouble—and you're going to write that it's just like my father and me.

J. M. – Well I think sometimes you want me to be like a father who can keep you from troubles.

S. – 'Don't bump my behind' says Big Bull to Warm-Behind Horse. And he says back, 'I've as much right to live in the land as you have.' Bull says, 'Then I have a right to keep my behind haven't I?' (The two twist round each other's noses as though they were wrestling.) These two are really angry with each other because they don't agree about their insides. Bull just happened to be there and that made Young Bull restless. I think Big Bull was a little bit right. What do you think, Dougie? Do you think Young Bull was right?

J. M. – I think Young Bull isn't too sure, because it's as though he were fighting for his father and against him too. Maybe he has mixed feelings about his father.

S. – Anyway Young Bull wins the fight. Now the men arrive with fanfare noises. Ooooh Pink Boy beats up one of them. Wham! These are really bad men and mean. Young Bull was sure scared. Now all the animals are going back to a silence and the troubles start again on Monday. A whole week of interesting shows. Into the stables. Tired, hungry, thirsty. Bad men all dead and everything going alright.

56th Session (Saturday 22.1.55)

When I read back the previous day's story game Sammy listens with his usual solemnity, but this time takes exception to the transference interpretations—perhaps because they deal more with the paternal aspects of the transference.

S.–No no! I don't ever think about you. I saw the most *exciting* thing of my life today and it wasn't *here*. I peeped in on my maid Ginette and I saw her behind! She was just undressing and I looked through the crack of the door. (He takes out the animals.) Today the bad men are going to take care of the animals. Young Bull—get out! I don't need you around the two bad men. The cattle come over looking for their master, that nice Pink Boy. They're wondering if he's going to get killed. Maybe they aren't really so bad. We shall find out! 'Oh, oh, five men against one isn't fair', says the Pink Boy. The men get him tied down. They shout things at him and whip him with a stick. Anyone would scream, but he's keeping his scream down. He's tied to the earth. He's going to get frightfully dirty. They've tied him to a tree, so tight it bleeds. But he's not hurt yet or hungry. The men all creep off and hide. It's night now. You're writing all my thoughts I hope? (I have in fact noted that Sammy thinks the punishment meted out to the Pink Boy is something like what he might expect the men to do if he wants to peep at women's behinds.) The poor animals cannot stay alone. A sad night's sleep! Now morning. The moon went down and the sun came out. But the days are not interesting now without the Pink Boy. At 12 o'clock at night all the animals stampede, with the bad men chasing them. Oh darling, all the animals jump from the mountains. All is silent except the birds and the trees and the breathing of the boy. He doesn't know a thing to do. Not a single thing. Poor boy getting iller and iller! More pains and terrible feelings, and weak and numb. Cold and shivering, and his clothes are getting dirty. 'Oh', he says, 'I don't want to die. I'm not going to bear it when the winter snow comes. If only I had a knife.' What's he going to do now Dougie? (He smiles at me as though we share a secret, and sings the Funeral March.) Warm-Behind Horse comes back and licks him on his cold arms. He's biting the rope with his teeth. Pink Boy says, 'Wonderful I'm getting loose.' And he falls on the horse with happiness. They run away together, and all the forest is gay.

57th Session (Monday 24.1.55)

Sammy arrives with lipstick on. He preens about, explaining meanwhile that he has obliged the maid to put it on him. He then becomes very agitated, saying it must all be washed off immediately, and that this operation must be verified in front of a glass. He starts screaming and thrashing around, too anxious to listen to anything I say. I give him some Kleenex and send him off to the bathroom. When he returns, his face scrubbed pink, he tells me that it would be terrible if ever his mother should know about the lipstick.

J. M. – You wouldn't want Mummy to think that you're copying her, sort of taking her place?

S. – No! Now write. You must write!!

Today the troubles start again. (Funeral March.) The Pink Boy calls the one who has the troubles. It's the buffalo, and oh darling, his great fat behind. A shining bare behind. Black Cow gets difficult again. Poor Buffalo feels ashamed of his trouble. (Funeral March. Sammy begins suddenly to yell, and makes the elephant charge into the table.) Oh oh look what's happening! Elephant is taking Pink Boy up, squealing he is, and he knocks him off the table. Oh darling, oh darling, what's going to happen now? (Under the table Sammy has removed the elephant's tusks. He then rolls onto the ground himself.) Come on, come and pick me up. Come on, Dougie.

J. M. – You'd like me to play games with you like the animals do together.

S. – Sh! Sh! Oh anyway, you're too mean to do a thing for me. (He picks himself up, and starts to sing theme from the Sorcerer's Apprentice.) The fight between these two continues. (Elephant and Warm-Behind Horse.) Elephant is losing. (In the heat of the battle Sammy lets one of the tusks fall to the ground. He pricks me in the arm with the other, wanting me to pick it up.) You're a bit lazy do you know?

J. M. – How did the elephant lose his tusks?

S. – The horse attacked him. There's a good big trouble! (The two tusks are carefully placed behind a tree.) That bad elephant, he really did the works. Now the elephant has kicked the bucket!! (He grins and gaily hums the Funeral March.) Now the search begins for the elephant's tusks, and whoever finds them will be the chief. Flicker has been chief up till now, with Pink Boy. The animals all stampede. Wild Horse finds a tusk. Who will find the other? The eyes have spied the tusk. It's the Black Cow! So these two will have to fight. Flicker has been thanked for the time he was president. Who's it going to be—Wild Horse or Black Cow for president? Who are you for Dougie?

J. M.–I'm not sure. What about you?

S.–Me? Oh I won't say because my side might lose and I wouldn't like that. Flicker's for Wild Horse. I'm always on Flicker's side so I'll be for Wild Horse too. Now whose side are you on? (Since I am pushed to choose I say that I will be on Flicker's side too. The animals are divided into two camps, and Wild Horse finally wins to the strains of the Hymn of Joy.) Black Cow slinks behind a tree, she's that sorry she can't be president, but she didn't want to kill him. Now for the buffalo's trouble. Oh boy, it's so long since I told a trouble I've forgotten how.

J. M.–This fight between Wild Horse and Black Cow seems to be a battle between mother and son to see who is going to take the father's place.

S.–Now Dougie, don't talk like that. It's just *luck* that Wild Horse won. Now guess this fellow's trouble (tapping the buffalo). Oh ladies, I'm going to tell (he pretends to cry but the panic of earlier sessions is not manifest). This young man here has a trouble, a hairy behind, so hairy that his BMs come out and it gets stuff all over. Now wait, I'm afraid I'll die if I don't make a happy ending. Then everyone will be fine and gay for the rest of his long life.

58th Session (Tuesday 25.1.55)

S.–I want to write down something different today, not a story. We're going to make up a medical form about our health.

(Sammy writes the following questionnaire himself and also fills in the answers given below.)

Now this is your form Dougie:

You are	5 ft 5 ins.
Healthy person	yes
Other? Appendix?.........	no
You have	32 teeth
Bad accidents..............	no
Bad sickness	'flu

Sammy then proceeds to a similar 'medical form' for himself:

You are   ....   4 ft 4 ins.
Teeth ....   26. 6 false. 2 gold.
Tonsils ....   no. Tongue operation was needed.
Health ....   Very healthy for certain. Insides going
fine these days.
Bad sicknesses ....   measles. 'Flu.
Bad accidents ....   Fell out of car. Hurt leg but no broken
bones.
Bad frights ....   Yes. As a little boy dreamed there was a
monster taking my father away who was very old.

Sammy is delighted with his forms, and files them importantly. He then dictates a second form which he says is to be a test, and which can be used for both of us simultaneously.

Big Test for Both of Us. The Story of Our Lives.
Dougie was 20 years old when she was born.
Sammy was born at 6 years.
Are you nice? Breath is bad but Sammy is fine.
Do you like yourself? (Sammy asks me what I wish to answer. I say yes.)

Sammy answers for himself 'So much that I faint.'

Do you have any breasts?
J. M. – Yes, two.
    S. – Hippopotamus ones. How are your intestines?
J. M. – Alright.
    S. – Very bad, mine.

Sammy then draws a series of hearts, and a circle with a cross in it. He adds some tubes to one of the heart drawings and tells me it is a heart with an aorta. He then draws a buttocks, and asks me to guess what it is and to give my answer in writing.

J. M. – (Writes) Is it somebody's bottom?
    S. – (Writes) Yes. Yours. (He surrounds my 'bottom' with large black crosses.)
J. M. – (Writes) Those crosses make me think there is something wrong with my bottom.
    S. – Yes.

114

J. M. – What about yours?

    S. – Like this. (He draws a long-shaped object in a straight line.)

J. M. – That looks more like a penis than a bottom.

    S. – No. It's a stick.

J. M. – So your bottom has a stick and mine doesn't?

    S. – (Writing) Go and see Dr Lubevese. Because you have a big head and a big gas pane and a bottom.

Under cover of the fantasy of playing the doctor Sammy faces the analytic situation in a more mature way. The nightmare in which a monster carries away his old father is a personification of Sammy's own aggressive wishes and oedipal fantasies. However, the whole of Sammy's analytic material up to the present suggests that behind this classical oedipal conflict is the imago of a devouring mother who wants to take possession of the father's penis and phallic power—in the same way that Sammy fears that the 'castrated' analyst wants to castrate him. While on the one hand Sammy is here demonstrating a projection of his own desire for possession of the father's penis he is at the same time expressing a regressive solution to an earlier desire—that of fusion with the mother—a defence against the anxieties of the classical oedipal situation. Experienced projectively as the devouring mother (or breasts) it is an attempt to beome the mother in order to control and possess her and so possess the power to attract the father's penis. The danger of this position is that it implies not only self-castration but annihilation of the self and the loss of ego identity. The primitive unconscious 'recognises' that in eating the lion's heart in order to possess his strength the lion is also destroyed. The desires directed towards both parents then engender profound guilt and anxiety of psychotic dimensions concerning the loss of the self and of the object world. Thus the drama begins when Sammy thinks of *breasts like a hippopotamus*. Immediately he feels his body is threatened and states that his intestines work badly—the internal objects are so destructive.

When the satisfaction and the fear aroused in him by the existence of his penis is interpreted, Sammy then turns to Dr Lebovici, an analytic father figure. But this homosexual refuge does not allow Sammy to escape from the fear of the 'big head' (the knuckle-head of former sessions), or the 'big gas pane' of intestinal omnipotence, all associated with the anxious 'breast-situation'.

59th Session (Thursday 27.1.55)

Sammy starts off reading the 'questionnaires'.

S.—You're a funny psychoanalyst!

J. M.–Why is that?

    S.–They're usually fierce like this (screws his face up in a grimace). They do that to frighten you. But I like to have a silly psychoanalyst. Do you like Dr Lebovici? I went to see him once. Don't you think he's better than you?

J. M.–You thought he was fierce?

    S.–Yes. I'm frightened of him.

J. M.–It's better to have a psychoanalyst who is frightening?

    S.–I wonder why I think he's better than you?

J. M.–Because he's a man?

    S.–Yes, perhaps. (He taps my chest with a pencil and giggles.)

J. M.–You think you'd be safer with him?

    S.–I'm going to work with him. I don't suppose he has any games like this. I'd be bored there. But just for the first few days I'd be frightened. Oh boy! I wish I was the psycho-analyst! You have a big trouble.

(He taps my breasts. I tell him that he can talk about my breasts but not hit me. Nevertheless he keeps trying to hit my chest, telling me all the while that it is a very great trouble, and how glad he is that he doesn't have any breasts.)

J. M.–You seem to be afraid of my breasts. You talk as though they could damage you.

    S.–Yes it's true. I know because my mother told me. Now just move off and let me take your chair.

J. M.–My breasts?

    S.–Ha! If you saw your breasts all bleeding what would you say?

J. M.–It seems you want to attack them, and take them for yourself.

    S.–Your breasts are bad. They could kill me!

(He jumps over towards me and tries to flick up my skirt, which I forbid. At the same time I say he can tell me what he imagines he would see.)

 S. – Telling is not amusing. I want to *see*.
J. M. – And what is it you want to see?
 S. – Up to your knees doesn't interest me. I want to see your behind.
J. M. – What do you imagine you would see?
 S. – Look, you'd be excited to see something you'd never seen before! I've never seen a *psychoanalyst's* behind. I must see women's behinds. I know they're just the same as men's, but I might even see a little bit of hair. Then I'll know what I'll [sic] look like.
J. M. – It sounds to me as if you expect to find I have a penis like you, and you don't have to want my breasts.
 S. – Oooooh, I'll never take my pants down and show you mine. My psychoanalyst in New York used to do it. And she used to lick my behind, while I was eating ice-cream. You wouldn't do that. You're too mean. Now please, just show me! You're that mean you are! Will you show me your bottom when I've finished my psychoanalysis?

Sammy spends the remaining minutes of the session trying to pull my skirts up by force. Remonstrance and interpretations having no effect, I tell him that the session is terminated. He quickly darts into his chair in order to announce the 'trouble' for today.

 S. – And his trouble for today is a fart-fart behind, a big behind. And he has a big bony behind but his troubles are all over. Everything is over.

(Sammy evades the breast-penis anxieties by concentrating solely on behinds.)

6oth Session (Friday 28.1.55)

 S. – What's wrong with you Today? (He looks at me guiltily then sits down and engages immediately in a long conversation about paintings he does at home and at school, and his wish to be an artist like his father. He keeps on with this line of talk, even repeating himself several times as though wishing to avoid quite other thoughts.)

S.–Yes, I want to be a painter I do. If God will help me, that is. He's part of everybody, so I might be helped by nature. I want to be famous though. Maybe I'll have my paintings put in the Louvre.

J. M.–So you might be even more famous than daddy?

S.–Oh I'm not going to try too hard! (There is a long silence, while Sammy looks at the toys, but doesn't make a move towards them.)

J. M.–Perhaps you find it hard to know what to do today after yesterday's talk about my breasts being so dangerous, and all the talk about bottoms.

S.–Oh yes. Oh boy! Am I glad I've got a bible! And a book of Rembrandt with my favourite painting in it. It's called Samson's Wedding Feast. (He begins to recount the Bible Stories from the beginning, but misses out Cain and Abel. I draw his attention to this.) Well, I hope I'll never do to my sister what he did. (He finally takes out the toys and begins placing them, moving them around silently, then explodes with rage because I am not writing.)

J. M.–I think you like me to write all the time because you find me dangerous if I'm not occupied.

(Sammy picks up a ball of plasticine and hurls it with full force at the animals, so that they all tumble. He sings wildly, switches into the Funeral March, then screams at me: 'Keep writing!' He picks up the pen himself and writes: 'All the animals are looking at the grate anoyanse. But haha ther is truble flying throu the air the thing that hit them was a grate BOMB. It was a lote a makeup thing. Dont worree.')

S.–Now the trouble is going to be told. Bull bumped his behind against Mother-Cow, their warm behinds together. They'll never do it again. And they stopped it for good and ever. P.S. The trouble was the bottoms that were together.

(All couples are bad especially when baby sisters may result from such unions.)

61st Session (Saturday 29.1.55)

After asking for yesterday's 'trouble' to be read back, Sammy tells a long story about visiting Ginette and her two-year-old son. Accord-

118

ing to Sammy this child is a miniature devil and has even been known to attack and cut someone once with a knife.

S. – Oh boy, I'll never go back to Ginette's place. It'll be bloody murder! Ya know, when she was working at our place today, I saw a bit of bare skin. Oh that Ginette—I'd really like to see her behind. When we went to the swimming pool yesterday together I asked if we could undress in the same cabin. But she wouldn't! Oh, and another terrible thing happened today – I saw a man lose his temper. Oh boy! I'm so glad I'm not . . . ah . . . oh no. I can't say it.

J. M. – Why, what would happen?

S. – I might die. Oh no. Not me. I'll never do what she did!

J. M. – (Now rather lost in the story.) Who, Ginette?

S. – No, silly. Eve in the Bible. (Bursts into strains of Grieg's Morning Song and starts to place his animals.) Now the story starts for today!

This horse has his ears flat—that means he's in a terrible temper. (Angry father-image.) All the others get out of the way. (Funeral March.) He bites everybody's tail. Now he attacks Mother Cow. He's biting on the udders! He's biting on the neck! Oh my, that horse is really mad. (The sexual father.) And the little Bull is suffering with fright, because the horse bit him too. (The father, angry with Sammy for peeping.) Wild Horse then attacks Donkey, biting hard, teeth gripping, ears flat. We're all going the same way home. Ah, that Wild Horse, it's his trouble. And the trouble shall be told at ten minutes to (i.e. at the end of the session). All the animals gather round to settle him down a bit. (Sings theme from Hall of the Mountain King.) Here comes the Pink Boy. He has a bottom ache and a belly ache but he's better. (Funeral March as Sammy rolls on the floor but in clearly mock anguish. In rolling around he tries to flick up my skirt.) Oh oh I'm suffering with fright. I shall be carried to a foreign land and thrown in an inkwell. I shall be thrown aside, cut to pieces . . . (he ad libs with his eye on his watch so that he can calculate the time required to tell the 'trouble' before the end of the session). And the trouble is—he has a real disease, not a make up one. It's called rabies, and that's why he was biting. Now his ears are forward again, and he has become better. But it was his fault he caught it! (I note down, to say to Sammy, that his peeping on Ginette's behind makes him expect trouble from an angry man.)

62nd Session (Monday 31.1.55)

Sammy tells about the fun he has on Sundays when he goes out with his father and they play races, the father in his car and Sammy running on foot. (These same outings and games had been reported by Sammy's father as a nightmare experience. Sammy's crazy and provoking behaviour makes him feel desperate. He changes his mind every few minutes about what he wants to do and where he wants to go, and the car-foot races form the only activity the father has discovered which will occupy Sammy for more than a few minutes. He said it gives him the impression of taking a little dog out for exercise.)

S.–Now these two cows are going to have a great fight. Ah, the Black Cow has run away. Write down my thoughts! (That I am still the Black Cow in Sammy's games.) She ran away because she was afraid of her behind. All the animals are frightened of their reflections today. (Funeral March as he starts to tap Flicker's behind.) What's wrong with you, Dougie? You better go and see Dr Lebovici! My word, Flicker is horrified that the chief would attack his own people. (J. M.–Is Dr Lebovici in this game?) Never you mind! Just keep on writing. And where is your Parker 51? What have you done with it? Why do you have that one?

J. M.–I've lost the other one.

S.–Well, it's not my fault!

J. M.–Why do you think it could be your fault? (He gets very very angry and apparently guilty because the pen is lost, and comes over to hit me.) You seem so cross about the loss of my pen, as though it were a part of me that's lost. It makes me think of all your worries about my insides as if you think I have a penis in there, and you would like me to give it to you.

S.–Dougie, you talk too much. I bet you talk a lot to your husband.

J. M.–You think I talk with my husband more than with you.

S.–Oh, if only you would talk about interesting things with *me*.

J. M.–So I do more interesting things with my husband?

S.–Yes. Tell me all about him. How *old* is he? (Sammy immediately brings up a ball of plasticine and fires it at me.)

J. M.–You're cross with me Sammy because of my husband who is a

120

man while you're still a young boy. And because you think I talk about interesting things with him and not with you.

S. – (Throwing all the toys at me.) Yes, I do! But *I'm* partly your husband!

Today Sammy projects on to me his anxiety about castration and disintegration. Perhaps he also thinks Dr Lebovici has taken back the pen I 'stole' from him. At the same time the chief attacks his own people—fathers might castrate their sons. While these castration themes are clearly linked to Sammy's jealousy of my husband, the pen-phallus probably also has a deeper meaning to him. Sammy gives me all his troubling thoughts and fantasies in the hope that I will organise them for him by writing them down. Just as the penis symbolises an organising agent, so he hopes to find some meaning through the welter of violence and fear in his stories, as they pass through my pen.

63rd Session (Tuesday 1.2.55)

S. – Now today's game is about this person. (He places a horserider on a pencil with a bit of plasticine and sings a theme from Beethoven's 2nd Symphony.) This is the ancient statue of the dead man. He died! (Funeral March.) He was one of the animal's masters a long time ago. A hurricane is flying over the country and all the animals are out looking at his statue. He was a bit strict with them. The ancient statue is rocking. All the animals gather round and they will make a new stand for him. (He mounts a second rider on a pencil and places him besides the first.) Now this chief will really stand up, no matter how the wind blows. The one on top is best, a little less than the worst. And the lower one here is not too good. But to be on the ancient statue is not too bad at all. Another of our friends shall be on the statue. Can you remember who died once Dougie? (He places the little calf on the statue to a tune from the Nutcracker Suite.) This statue shall be called the Tower of Babel. I hope this tower is blessed, so people are good to it. (It has now become a highly complicated structure balanced upon the plasticine pot.) Oh I'm really proud of it. Would you make a little sketch of it for me? (He comes over as though to assist, but profits from this move to throw my skirt up and tries to grab at me underneath the skirt. I take hold of his wrists to stop him.) You're not going to slap me are you?

J. M. – No. But I'm not going to let you do that either. (Sammy struggles free and starts grabbing at my clothing.)

S. – Oh, oh, I've found ... I've found ...

J. M. – Don't worry Sammy. I'm *not* going to let you put your hands inside my clothing.

Sammy seems calmed by the reassurance that I will always prevent this kind of acting out. He returns to the statue and begins modelling little balls to add to it, muttering about them as though they were little bits of me he has managed to annex.

S. – There now Dougie. I got it anyway and now it's safer. This statue is really famous for its three balls. There's the entrance. (More balls are added to the entrance.) Oooh I think this tower is going to get ever more famous. Famous for what it is. The best tower of all, says me.

> The prohibition of Sammy's desire to act out no doubt fostered his pleasure in building his tower, and it is just at that moment that he has the idea of adding the first series of three balls. He later adds three more to the 'entrance'. I seems to me that he here symbolises 'making it safer' in two ways, first by giving me the 'breast-testicles' without which I am dangerous to his penis, and second he introduces in this way a paternal element into the transference. This is perhaps all the more necessary, since in this game oedipal rivalry and masculine identification have to some extent ended in failure. Father and little dead calf are both on the ancient statue, that is, little calf can be with the father when both are dead. I think the 'Tower of Babel' also represents Sammy's own confusion, and his tangled relationship to the maternal imago. He needs the father and the phallus in order to make things clearer.

Interview with Sammy's teacher (1.2.55)

Mme Dupont had requested this interview herself and Mrs Y was in agreement. I gathered she was feeling anxious about her new pupil and I myself was interested to hear how Sammy behaved in the school situation.

Sammy first joined the little class in September, 1954 about the time he began his analysis. He was terrified of everybody and every new object he saw, and at the same time his behaviour was quite intolerable. He missed no occasion for provoking and irritating Mme Dupont. He could do no school-work of any kind and every play activity ended in complete failure and an outburst of violence from Sammy.

In view of all his previous years of total scholastic failure and this first bleak month of seeking contact with him, Mme Dupont despaired of getting anywhere. However, she found that when he was anxious she could bring him back to normal by rocking him like a baby and feeding him with a baby bottle, this latter being frequently requested by him. When he was violent she discovered that smacking him had an immediate calming effect. Towards the middle of November Sammy was able to concentrate for short periods, sufficient to make some beginning with learning. His conversation, however, still did not make sense. He never once spoke of anything real he had seen or done, only imaginary things. During December he suddenly started to make astonishing progress and in the last three months has covered the equivalent of three years' normal school work.

Recently Sammy asks endless questions about Mme Dupont's private life. In particular he wants to know if she washes herself thoroughly. He is capable of asking this question fifty times in a day. Monsieur Dupont who suffers from a heart condition is also the subject of many questions. Sammy says he is afraid of him, speculates on his death, etc. These aspects of Sammy's behaviour no longer worry her. Also she is encouraged by his surprising progress, even though he has to learn like a baby, everything being turned into a game. In addition, he now talks about real events from time to time, more like a normal child and his comportment in general is less bizarre. She is beginning to think he is very intelligent.

64th Session (Thursday 3.2.55)

S. – The trouble with you is that you never laugh. Everyone in the world laughs but you. At lunch time they all laughed today because I told funny stories. I said I once went to a school where you got 25 hits if you batted an eyelid. Now what would you have said?

J. M. – I'd have said that you must think real school is a very frightening place.

S. – Oh but no one believed me. Now where's my tower? Oh me, oh men it's going to get frightening if it gets too tall. The real tower of Mabel she's called and they thought it touched the heavens. It won't matter if mine does that (Nutcracker Suite). Oooh men, if I get too famous what, oh men, will you say? You'll get mad if I get it too high. (Looking at me.) It's getting bothering, Dougie. I'm getting more and more worried about it. Will you let me go on doing it?

J. M. – You think I won't be pleased if you do exciting things like this tower?

S. – Yes. I'd like to make something fantastic, real fantastic. Something enormous, big and gorgeous. But if I make it too good . . . oh you! You're spoiling all my fun. Oh fuckins! You're spoiling it, you're going to say, 'Now Sammy that will do'. I know you're going to knock it down and spoil all my fun!

J. M. – Really, Sammy, you seem to want me to spoil your fun. It's as though you think I am jealous of it.

S. – Do you remember the time I threw things at you?

J. M. – That's when you were concerned with those thoughts about my husband and me together?

S. – Yes. Did you like that? And if I hit you really hard again with the chessman would you like that? What would you do?

J. M. – I wouldn't like it much. But I think you really want to know if it's safe for us to be here together and to talk about all these exciting thoughts.

S. – Could I just pretend to hit you and you pretend to hit me back? (He comes over at that moment and touches me very lightly on the cheek with his little finger, then asks me to do exactly the same to him which I do.) Oh, Dougie, look it doesn't do anything! See, you're still alive!

J. M. – Yes and so are you.

S. – Now my tower can be great (he continues building it up) and then, Dougie, *you* will sing the Funeral March. This is just what it will be like when my analysis is finished, like I don't have any troubles any more. (He looks suddenly anxious in face of this upsurge of positive feeling.) But you've still got a trouble—your knuckle-head! Go and see Dr Lebovici. He'll fix you up. He'll . . . he'll . . . give your head a great big bash! (Sammy thinks that if he gets well I shall fall ill.)

Sammy then does a drawing entitled 'Dougie with 42 ears' and retitles it 'Dougie's Knuckle-head'. At the bottom of the page he writes, 'I would like if you would be so kind and kiss me', and he brings this missive round for me to read, presents his cheek and says, 'O.K. let's go!' I am a little nonplussed at this approach, knowing how much he needs to feel that his love feelings like his hate feelings are not destructive; at the same time I fear an uncontrollable outburst of anxiety on his part. I tell him this and give him a little kiss on the upturned cheek which he is still patiently presenting. He shows no terror but pleasure, as with the 'hits'.

S. – Now please, Dougie, note *all* the thoughts to tell me tomorrow.

After the session I noted, 'Today Sammy wanted to know what things are safe and what are dangerous. Like when he was building the tower and wanted it to get bigger and higher, and was so sure I would spoil his fun. I think he really wanted to know whether I would approve of his being so interested in his penis and making it bigger and higher. And later on he needed the hitting game to see if we could touch one another without either of us getting damaged. Sammy worries about angry thoughts doing damage too. Then he wanted the same game with the kiss, to see if it was dangerous. But all these frights also made Sammy want Dougie to be a bit like a father too. He thinks Dr Lebovici would be like a strong father-person who will keep both Dougie and Sammy in place.'

Throughout this session (beginning with the made-up story about the slaps he got in school) Sammy has been seeking the prohibition of a highly eroticised contact, this latter representing a double danger. On the genital level, he cannot but imagine that his tower will be smashed and his fun spoiled, and later 'Dougie's knuckle-head' has to be seen to by Dr Lebovici. But in his pre-genital fantasy the dangerous mother image (the Tower of Mabel) threatens him with her hidden phallic attributes and her envy of his penis. Nevertheless he plucks up the courage to play out the aggressive exchange which the fantasied primal scene represents for him. At this point he introduces a paternal figure, and pictures, as it were sadistic intercourse between the two analysts.

65th Session (Friday 4.2.55)

After having yesterday's session read out, Sammy remarks that he is very pleased with it, and in particular the ending, where I write down his 'thoughts'. He then asks if he could have a glass of milk, which I interpret to him as a need for reassurance.

S. – But look, when you go into a café you don't go in with the thought that they are to be good fathers to you. And you're probably thinking at the bottom of your head that when I want milk it's got something to do with those breasts popping out. Yes?

J. M. – If you say so, it probably has. You want milk. And at the same time you know that you're not very pleased to get it, as though it also meant something else.

S. – You know, Dougie, something funny is happening. I'm getting tired of the Fifth Symphony these days too. (This has always been his favourite record. He would listen to it for hours on end.) Is it bad that I like listening to music so much?

J. M. – Perhaps you ask me that because it's connected in your mind with all the games you play here to music . . . the fart-fart and all that.

S. – Do you touch your husband's behind?

J. M. – You would like to know more about what goes on with my husband and myself, like with your mother and father. And it's probably got something to do with your thoughts about me too.

S. – But *do* you? Would you touch his behind if he wanted it?

J. M. – You keep talking about behinds. I wonder if that's because it's less frightening than talking about our fronts?

S. – Oh, I know, I know. They put their penises together. I know that. But is it alright to touch behinds? (So saying, Sammy leaps from his chair, rushes at me and fights to pull up my skirt.)

J. M. – Sammy you know perfectly well that I'm not going to allow you to pull up my skirt. I think you want me to get angry with

126

you and forbid you even to talk about these things. I know that these ideas are frightening to you too sometimes, so it's important for us to talk about them.

S.–Alright. Tell me, have you a penis?

J. M.–No. This you know.

S.–Well, well! I want to *see*. (This time he becomes really aggressive and has to be firmly stopped. He listens to no interpretations touching his anxiety etc., and only the threat of terminating the session has any effect.)

S.–Would you think it was awful if children touched behinds?

J. M.–Why, what makes you think of that?

S.–Well, once I was at a little girl's place, and we went to the bathroom and touched bottoms. Then the two fathers came in and said we mustn't do that. That it was very babyish. I want to see yours. Well, if you won't, show me a drawing!

J. M.–Supposing you make a drawing of what you expect to find.

S.–Oh yes. I know, we'll both do one. (He quickly supplies us both with pencils and paper.) Now do front and back view!

Sammy's front-view woman has a large mass of pubic hair and distinctly feminine contours. The back view looks markedly masculine and there is a suggestion of a penis drawn between the legs. They are labelled respectively, 'Dougie's Front' and 'Dougie's Bottom' and under the latter, 'Oh man am I so happy to see Dugys BOTTOM'. I make schematic undetailed drawings which don't please Sammy very much but he is delighted with his own. I'm also pleased he is able to control his desire to act out the voyeuristic and aggressive impulses which arise each time he is anxious about sexual differences and primal scene fantasy, and to accept the drawings as a satisfying substitute.

66th Session (Saturday 5.2.55)

Sammy immediately asks to see the drawings, and expresses delight at this new form of gratification.

S.–Oh boy! I'd love to come in one day and find you all naked. I'd kiss your breasts and rub my head in your crotch and pat your behind and press myself against your breasts. Oh boy, oh boy! (There follows a spate of questions such as: Do you pat you husband's behind? Does he ever want to pat yours? What do you say?

J. M.—It seems to me you're jealous of my husband.

S.—Would you *ever* let me pat yours? (in a pleading anxious tone.)

J. M.—No. But that doesn't mean we can't talk about it.

S.—If I ever have a wife who pats my behind or wants me to pat hers, I'll slap her till her face is green!! I'll never stand for that!

J. M.—You think it's very naughty to want that.

S.—Yes. You mustn't do it. Dougie, do you ever look at yourself in the mirror?

J. M.—If I want to, yes.

S.—But do you look at your bottom? At the bottom hole?

J. M.—You think that's naughty too?

S.—Oh I don't do it! It's very babyish. You'll never see my penis. If ever you see my penis, oh boy, I'll be murdered!

J. M.—How's that?

S.—Your big bosoms would murder me. Oh my! I don't know if you should see my penis or not? (He ponders this as though it is a question which has to be decided upon. It seems that the envied breasts will destroy his penis.) No. And I'd better not draw myself when I'm on the toilet seat. I wonder if you like yourself when you're all naked.

J. M.—You think there's something bad about being naked too?

S.—Oh yes, I'll say!

J. M.—You think it's dangerous like drawing or showing your penis?

S.—Oh boy, yes! Now just a few minutes before the end, let's leave enough time to draw what I look like. (He says this in almost the same words which he used formerly to tell the 'troubles'.)

He sets to immediately and draws his front and back views, and demands that I do likewise. In his back view he is going towards the bath. The front view represents Sammy in the bath. He hums and haws over this drawing because he does not know how to draw his penis in effectively. He wishes it to be represented accurately, and, at the same time, to be much in evidence. Once finished he is very pleased with the results. He looks with great interest at my efforts.

S.—Oh I'm much prettier than that. I'm not so tall and skinny and my penis isn't so pointed. Look, I'll draw it for you.

128

(He draws a belly with a pair of legs and a carefully drawn penis. He then decides to pin all the drawings on the wall. This done, he takes up a pencil, taps his 'penis' and my 'breasts', and hums the Funeral March.)

67th Session (Monday 7.2.55)

Sammy recounts that a boy on a bicycle ran into him yesterday, and Sammy's father became extremely angry with the boy in question.

S. – It's a great shame I have to come here, because of all my boy-friends. Well, it's not really true that I have lots of boy-friends, but I *had* lots in New York.

J. M. – You like to think of your father who protects you, and of the boy-friends in New York, so you can feel more at ease with me here.

S. – It's because I'm really afraid of your behind. Women's behinds are more frightening than men's. (I try to lead him to expand on this idea, but he passes to other preoccupations which are always interwoven in his mind with these themes.) Supposing you died of starvation, how would you like it? I wouldn't mind because I'm different. I have a — (he points to his penis).

J. M. – You could feed yourself with it?

S. – (With great certainty.) Oh yes. Just look in the mirror yourself and find out.

J. M. – Find out what?

S. – Would you please look in the mirror for me tonight? Please. That'll prove that you're a good person.

J. M. – You mean if I have a penis I'm a good person?

S. – Sometimes I wonder if you're a bad person.

J. M. – What's a bad person?

S. – Someone who bites their own penis. Ah but you, you bite your breasts instead.

J. M. – So I'm a bad person.

S. – Oooh I'm really afraid you're going to bite my penis. (Half joking, half panic-stricken tone in his voice. He is on the point of throwing something at me.)

J. M. – You seem to think penises and breasts are much the same thing, as if you think they're dangerous for one another and can both be eaten, too.

129

S.–Oh no. I don't have any thoughts like that. I say, could we have another hitting game like the other day? (He comes over and tries to whack me with a wad of plasticine stuck on a pencil. He gallops over my chair, seeking physical contact by these haphazard means, then tries to dislodge me from my chair because he would like me to sit on his knees. This I refuse, and insist that he return to his own chair.)

S.–What would you do if you fell into the toilet just after doing BMs? And why won't you sit on my knees? Ginette does. And my teacher too. So why not you? (He begins to draw, hiding the drawing with his hand.) Oh am I glad I don't have a behind like you. Yours is a cold behind. Ooooooh if you saw what I'm drawing I wonder what you'd say. Hey write! Keep on writing or you'll be punished.

(I have occasionally managed to get Sammy to talk to me without the reassurance of seeing me writing but this never lasts long without his becoming uncontrollably anxious. He makes three drawings, the first entitled 'Dougie's big behind' the second 'Dougie with a thin behind'. He covers this drawing with his hands, and later scribbles all over and around it. The third drawing is called 'Dougie going to the toilet'. This last drawing shows a water closet seen from above, and suspended over it is a large dark mass.)

S.–Do you remember the time I hit you? I'm glad I did that, otherwise you might bite my penis off.

J. M.–You must be very frightened of me, Sammy. You have to hit me to protect yourself.

S.–(Air of great seriousness.) I thought you'd get all these frights away. You're a psychoanalyst. That's all the frights I have. I've told you every one of them. Do you think you'll get them all away? Oh, there's another one. But I don't like to say it. (Shuddering.) It's about your insides. I keep thinking of your intestines popping out, and all your tripes and kidneys . . . etc. Oh Dougie, we must get all these frights away.

68th Session (Tuesday 8.2.55)

Sammy arrives once more with lipstick and rouge on, but on this occasion he is in no way anxious about it.

130

S. – Did you look at your behind? Do you often look at it? At your bosoms? Ooooh, they look awful, I can tell you. I feel real sorry for you, since I have a penis. It's much better than a bosom. (He begins to construct a plasticine tower.) Ooooh if it gets too high, the President of the United States will get after me. But you must go to Dr Lebovici because you have a bosom. He's a bit more like me, with a penis. Oooooh I'm frightened of your bosoms. I'm no better than I was. It's a good shame. You're such a dull psychoanalyst. I wish you could help me with my problems. But you don't say anything. you don't even care about my troubles. I don't care about your bosom! I'm only caring about my penis! You should be a dictator, you never like to stay in your own pants. You know—you're a dull person! And you have a big behind! (Singing.) A trouble is flying through the air. And it's your fat behind. It's quite different from a man's; a man's behind has dark skin and that's stronger. I like mine better than yours because I have a penis and you don't. D'ya know that? Hey, don't you stop writing.

J. M. – You talk as though you are afraid I might have a penis all the same, and a dangerous one at that.

S. – Well, you might. But you haven't. Well, but you might want one.

J. M. – Afraid I want yours?

S. – Because it's so easy to take my penis away. And to eat it.

J. M. – You really believe that?

S. – Yes yes! My mother said it was true. Dougie, it's true.

J. M. – You seem to want me to believe it, anyway.

S. – But if all the newspapers said so, and if all the hospitals said it was true, you would believe it then. And if one day you saw someone cutting off my penis, then you'd know.

J. M. – Sounds as if you would rather get rid of your penis sometimes, than have all these worries connected with it.

S. – If all the people in the world came to take off my penis what would you do? If Dr Lebovici came and did it? What would you do if your behind was bitten off? And what would you do if rains of BMs came down? If the doctor came to say I would die the next day in great pain what would you do? I want your behind! I would pat it and kiss it and rub it and hug it. And what would you do if one day you were paralysed all

131

over? (During all this one-way conversation, Sammy has been struggling to make his tower, but constructs it in such a way that it is practically impossible for it to remain upright. He keeps trying, patiently, to make it stand, but I have the impression that he wants it to fail as a structure.)

Perhaps as a consequence of having expressed so vividly in the last session his sexual fantasies, Sammy today oscillates between a masculine oedipal position and a homosexual one, both of which prompt him to think of a male analyst. He is uncertain whether I am a dull-person-without-a-penis or whether I am, on the contrary, safe from castration and better off that way.

69th Session (Thursday 10.2.55)

S. – I had a dream but I won't tell you. You wouldn't tell me what the last one meant. Let's read what we talked about last time.

(I give him a summary of his many questions and tell him that I have the impression that he thought it was better to get rid of his penis than to face all the worries and frights it caused him.)

S. – Well there's something else exciting. I hope the Seine will overflow! (According to the day's news there is a strong possibility that Sammy's wish will materialise.) What would you do if the water in the Seine comes right over the head of the Zouave Statue, etc. etc. (Sammy continues to invent ever more dangerous or absurd situations. He finally arrives at the following.) What would you do if the water reached the top of the Eiffel Tower?

J. M. – Well what would you do?

S. – Oh I'd take a boat and put my parents in it, and lots to eat, and we'd swim around in the boat for a long time, and after that we'd all just drown.

70th Session (Friday 11.2.55)

Sammy continues to talk excitedly about the Seine (still rising) and then thinks of Moses and the drowning of the Egyptians.

S. – Oh I love that Bible. I gave a long sigh when I heard how strict the Pharaoh was with those people. Supposing you were living then and you had me in analysis, and you saw the Egyptians whipping me, what'd you say?

J. M. – What would you like me to say?

S. – Well suppose you saw 600 people all rushing against me what would you do?

J. M. – I would say right now that you want me to protect you against all the scary things you like thinking up for yourself. (Sammy managed to think up many other such situations of exquisite danger which I did not note down, until such time as he himself became aware I was not occupied in writing.)

S. – And what would you say if a man came in and said that either you have to die or me? Tell me, do you like the Bible? Now I'm going to draw your flat with water all round it. Now, how would you get in? (Sings the Funeral March.) I keep wondering if you like your behind. Do you look at your bottom, your appendix, your tonsils . . . etc. Oh your knuckle-head worries me! What would you say if you saw a lady all naked in your room here?

J. M. – Well I'd say there must be some reason why Sammy thinks of a naked lady sitting here.

S. – Write my thoughts Dougie! And don't say I'm scared!! You might *think* it worries me, but it's not true.

J. M. – You once said you'd like to find me all naked when you came in, and people can be scared of things they say they would like.

S. – Well uh, if you came in and found lots of people all crowded in here suddenly what would you say?

J. M. – I'd say, 'Get out, people, or you will bother Sammy.'

S. – (Who finds this uproariously funny.) And if one of them made a smell—don't worry, I'm not scared of anything—what would you say?

J. M. – That that will bother Sammy, and that he really wanted to make the smell himself.

(Sammy is again utterly delighted; he draws the naked lady, himself and me, and writes a dialogue underneath).

Sammy sees lady: Oh, oh!!
Dougie: I don't like that!

Naked Lady: Don't worry. I won't do any harm.
Sammy: Oh sakes! You get out of here.
And then Sammy came in and whipped them till their behinds were
bleeding. (End of dialogue.)

>   S. – What would you do if a man went peepee on your floor. What
>   if he went peepee in your face? And if he went in the toilet and
>   you opened the door and found water up to the roof?
> J. M. – I'd say you would like to drown the people in this house with
>   your peepee.
>   S. – Oh boy!

Sammy then wants us to read his dialogue with the Naked Lady.
We read it each taking various roles. He makes up a 'second act'
which he doesn't write down, in which crowds of people pour into
the room, and all are naked; Sammy treats them with great ferocity
for coming in in such numbers, and in such nudity. He massacres a
fair proportion of them in varied sadistic ways and the rest are
disposed of by being pushed out of the flat where they all tumble
down the stairs. Along comes a big strong character who knocks them
all into a ditch and battens them down. 'And they all dieeeeeed'
squeals Sammy with great excitement. As he goes out he pleads that
I write a *happy* ending to this story.

>   Sammy clearly wants to recreate for me his imagined scenes
>   of castration and of intercourse in which he wants me to
>   participate but at the same time he wishes me to protect him
>   from them too. This is the same conflict of desire and fear
>   which he has shown so often in his former anal fantasies.

71st Session (Saturday 12.2.55)

In recapitulating yesterday's session, Sammy finds it suddenly
necessary to go to the toilet when we come to the bit about Moses
drowning the Egyptians. I point out to Sammy, along with the other
interpretations, the importance that urethral fantasies would seem to
have for him; he listens contentedly as always, and nods his agreement.

>   S. – Well I think now we'll have a different story. Now this is a
>   boat, I'm drawing you and me in it. See? But here is some-

thing sticking out (it turns out to be the top of the Eiffel Tower poking up above the water). Then the waters go down (a second and then a third drawing show larger and larger portions of the Eiffel Tower). And then it comes to pass that the sun gets hot and the water goes into rain, and then the water level starts to go up again. What would you say if it went billions of miles into the air?

(Then follows a series of such drawings, and the final drawing shows the Pont Alma and the water of the Seine washing over the feet of the Zouave, the statue at the foot of the bridge pillars.)

It was notable in this session that Sammy did not insist that I write down his stories, and also tolerated that I reply from time to time to his fantasies without his getting either aggressive, or terrified, or so involved in the relationship with me as to be unable to continue with his train of thought.

72nd Session (Monday 14.2.55)

S. – If I came very late what would you do? What would you think had happened to me?

Sammy continues to put many questions of this kind with great insistence, and my attempts to elicit his fantasy lead nowhere. I point out to him that he seems to need to reassure himself that I am capable of protecting him from any dangers that might befall him either here with me, or elsewhere.

S. – Well, what would you say if your *husband* got killed?
J. M. – Perhaps you are wondering what it would be like if you were my husband?
S. – Well . . . ah well . . . well let's say your husband died of a sickness. What would you do? Would I still come to see you? You know, you might be busy cleaning it up and so on. Oh, by the way, my parents say I might be going to a special school in America.
J. M. – Did your parents say this?
S. – You ask them! Now I'm going to draw things. See, those are all bridges.

J. M. – Are the bridges because you were thinking about a separation between us if you should go back to America?

S. – (With an air of great surprise.) I say can you tell people's *thoughts* from their drawings? (He pulls out a series of drawings he had made of the Seine rising, flooding, ebbing and so on.) What about these? Why did I do them?

I tell Sammy that he is intrigued by the imminent flooding of the Seine like everyone else, but that in addition it probably interests him because it is water. I recall his fantasies of urethral potency and the water in the toilet which would go up to the roof etc. Sammy is utterly delighted with this long interpretation.

S. – You promise these are my thoughts? Promise, Dougie? Hey, let's do some more.

He draws a chair, and a table with a jar on it. On being questioned he says the jar contains plasticine or clay, he thinks. I remark that the drawing is an exact reproduction of his chair and the table between us, complete with pot of plasticine. Sammy seems literally astonished by this rather banal remark.

S. – But I wasn't thinking of that at all. Oh this is fun. I was trying to make a drawing where you wouldn't see anything

He then draws a boy. Sammy says it is an ordinary boy who is just keeping his hands up in the air. He then draws a hallway, with a staircase leading down from it, and an arrow pointing to a closed door. He says there is a secret where the arrow points. The disposition of the hall, stairs and door corresponding exactly to my consulting room etc., which I point out to him. Again he is quite amazed. He follows this with a similar drawing, but this time the arrow is double-headed, and the second arrow points clearly in the direction of the toilet. I tell Sammy that perhaps there is a secret to tell which has to do with the toilet.

S. – Oh boy! Well what about this one. Here's a little horse that was very hungry. He came to this stall and was delighted to find a bucket. He was sure he would find food to eat, but there wasn't anything at all.

J. M. – I wonder if that's got something to do with you and me, and your disappointment at not finding everything you wanted here with me.

136

When I tell Sammy that our time is up for today he rapidly draws a chain of heads linked by one continuous line. (Fig. 2.)

J. M. – It looks to me as though this drawing is a way of not separating and saying goodbye!

Sammy was highly pleased with his session and with the possibility of studying his 'thoughts' in a new way. He did not at any point ask me to note down his words!

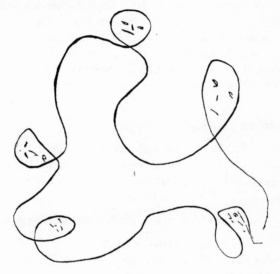

FIG. 2

Interview with Sammy's parents 14.2.55

Without my realising it, Sammy had announced the reason for this visit requested by Mr and Mrs Y two days ago. They came to discuss a vacancy in an American Special School for psychotic children. A year ago, before the move to Paris, they had made inquiries. Now they are undecided about accepting this offer which has arrived unexpectedly. They would like to keep Sammy with them in Paris but are worried about schooling since he seems to be making great progress recently. Nevertheless, he is more and more difficult at home, never satisfied and constantly tormenting and irritating his mother. Also he continues to embarrass visitors. He can for the first time in his life now play alone and also go for walks on his own. But like everything else he carries this independence to excess, stays out for hours, or when at home will paint for hours and only in oils. Thus his progress makes his behaviour even more intolerable in his parent's eyes. Also he no longer listens to music as he used to do.

My impression is that Mrs Y, accustomed to the limitations of Sammy's personality, is becoming anxious as his world enlarges. She may feel resentful of this and be punishing him unconsciously by wanting to send him to a boarding school. Mr Y is wholly opposed to the project, and draws attention to Sammy's marked school improvement and the fact that his teacher believes him capable of attending ordinary school one day. Mrs Y thinks the teacher exaggerates the improvement in Sammy's work. In any case no definite decision will be made until the Director has seen Sammy, which will be in a month's time.

73rd Session (Tuesday 15.2.55)

S. – Tell me again all the thoughts in my drawings.

J. M. – You know, Sammy, I can't see your thoughts. But the drawings might help us both to understand better the thoughts you have in the back of your mind.

Sammy then draws 'A man in a hardware store who fixes things'.

J. M. – What do you think it might mean?

S. – He's made a table and now he has to fix it up. I want it to be a bit puzzling for you but not too much.

J. M. – Maybe I'm the hardware man and you want me to fix you up?

S. – That's it. Now I know what the next one is going to be. There, it's a young vine, all beautiful and growing.

J. M. – That must be you I think.

S. – Well now here's a picture of an 'Ideal Boy'.

J. M. – Is that you too?

S. – Oh no, not me! This boy is twelve, he has a little dog and lives in the country with his parents. He loves them both, and he loves each of them just the same. He never goes to school, but he hates always having to stay at the house because he gets bored with nothing to do. When he's big he will write books. He reads 'Tom Sawyer' in English. He's very well brought up, a real thoroughbred. He was just born like that.

138

And he will live a very long time. You see it's not me. I won't live long, I'm much too bad. You know, I don't behave well. Now let me make another drawing. There are two old witches here, each with her own house, and in between the two there is an object. We don't know what it is. Sometimes this object is high up, like that, and sometimes it falls right down. These old witches are awful. They yell all the time. And they get on very well together. They're both so terrible, that's why. And they get hold of people and throw them into inkwells, and tear them up.

J. M. – I wonder if those two old witches aren't your mother and me? You know she came to see me the other night to talk about you. Perhaps the 'object' that goes up and down has something to do with you.

S. – My penis, that's what it is!

J. M. – It could be that you think we want to attack your penis, and stop you being a boy.

S. – Here's a treasure locked in a box. It's not a penis. If the thought that comes out is that it's a penis, well it's wrong. It's a very special treasure put there by a wicked wizard. At the back of his head he's really very nice, but he doesn't know it. He's proud of the treasure in this box. Perhaps it shall be won by the pretty prince. But you have to know how to get at it, to open it.

J. M. – Whatever do you think it can be?

S. – Maybe the next drawing will tell us. Here's something all smashed up. It's all in bits, and it isn't my penis. It's something that could have been very useful, but people have done this.

The drawing in question is perfectly round, and the lines indicating its breaking have been drawn all over it.

J. M. – It's a round thing.

S. – I know perhaps it's breasts! They're useful aren't they? Now this next drawing is a little elephant. He's very nice and very cheeky.

74th Session (Thursday 17.2.55)

S. – Now let me look at yesterday's drawings. Ooooh boy, I'm going to do some more. This is a whole city. These are the

139

houses in a town called Hawkon. The people there speak Hawkonish. This window-cleaner is sort of quiet. He washes his teeth every day and his face, and takes baths. Jolly and chubby he is.

Sammy then draws 'A little bit of smoke, not a volcano, coming out of the ground. The smoke is warm and it makes a sound as it comes out. Once the smoke got so unusual that it made patterns everywhere, like this.' I give Sammy an interpretation along the lines of his anal interests and the power and fascination they have for him. He is delighted and goes over it all himself, saying that it was funny he hadn't thought of it but he is sure that it is right.

The third drawing is described by Sammy as 'a broken chair in the middle of the desert, with nothing on it but a cushion. The chair used to be useful but now it's old and thrown away. It was getting so ugly that nobody wanted it.'

> S. – Whatever does it mean? Oh, I know! I know all by myself! The people who threw this chair away are like me. They all like good and comfortable things. I'm like that. I liked to drink warm milk sitting in a chair when I was little. Maybe it's got to do with bosoms too. I would feel safe, and would like it if someone would pay attention to me, all quiet and nice. But this chair is bad and old and all the things I don't want. Oh the little thought! I found it all by myself.

The fourth drawing is 'A statue of Jesus with people humming the Funeral March all round, and saints and nuns praying.'

J. M. – Why the Funeral March?
> S. – It means God. And it has to do with punishment too.

The fifth drawing: 'A car with bad people in it. They're pushing a little boy into a car—no, it's a little girl, no it's both. At the end of the road there is smoke. You never know what's at the end of the road, ladies!'

The sixth drawing: 'This is the princess's magic finger pointing to something. She's so famous her finger sparkles. We don't know what she's pointing at, but don't worry. If it gets too famous her finger gets famous too. Now here is the thing that is happening to her finger, but we don't know what it is.'

Seventh drawing: 'A bunch of people all see this thing flashing by in the sky. Bright lights like lightening as they stare, and it makes such a racket. Whatever is going on? What can it be?

Sammy begins singing the Funeral March. I interpret his drawing as possibly being related to his interest in primal scene fantasies sometimes frightening to him, but which make him want to stare and to listen.

> S. – Oh, but I'm not frightened of that any more. My parents can do what they like. But I'll put a cross beside it, because it's a very interesting thought.

Still singing the Funeral March loudly Sammy makes his eighth drawing.

> S. – Know what? It's a grave this time. But whose or what, that's what I want to know. There's me and my father and my mother and my sister beside it. And there's you, Dougie, just so you'll know it's not you who's in the grave.
>
> J. M. – Maybe you are afraid of having such thoughts about me?
>
> S. – But I don't get angry with you any more. Still it's all getting very frightening inside of me.

Ninth drawing. This drawing shows a large face with a cross over its mouth.

> S. – Oooh! This drawing is very spooky, there's a big fat, chubby cross on his mouth. I made it frightening. It's called the Face. It's not you. It's very important to see what he's thinking of inside his head. There's a dead person beside a grave. It's the son that's dead and his mother is there crying. Now tell me the thought, Dougie, please?
>
> J. M. – Somehow I think you did have an idea of me all the same when you drew the face. And maybe you're afraid of what might come out of my mouth and that it could bring about your death. I think this drawing has something to do with you being afraid of your own dangerous thoughts and this leads to your thinking I might have dangerous thoughts towards you. And of course there is this idea about going to a school in America.
>
> S. – Ah ha! Ah ha! (He chants the Funeral March.) Here's the Jewish star, and a cross beside it and a regular star. And here's a cross on a person that's not you. He's famous in a way, he's a sort of a ghost.

141

The series of drawings reveal a dramatic progression over which, however, Sammy retains a fair control. From this point of view his own interpretation of his fantasy of the chair, broken and abandoned in the desert, is important in terms of the impending separation suggested by the special school, and Sammy needs now to find the 'thoughts' for himself. Maybe I am the old chair that will have to be thrown away. This would make it easier for him to face leaving.

The tragic death themes also stimulated by the threatened separation begin to appear with the fourth drawing in which Jesus is represented on the cross. The fifth drawing provides a link between the aggression which leads to mortal danger and the anal fixations which were interpretated in the second drawing.

The interpretation of the primal scene is accepted by Sammy with reservations, and he demonstrates the extent to which he is now able to control his anxiety during this stage of the treatment. However, this reanimates his anxiety in the transference. First, he pictures himself before a tomb; then we have a typical illustration of the mode of thought peculiar to him—the head whose mouth wears 'a fat, chubby cross'. Dougie-Magic Face is going to die. Finally the face becomes the tomb itself. For the first time we see some of the protective magic-thinking associated with Sammy's singing the Funeral March wherever his fantasies are particularly violent and destructive, or sad and disturbing.

75th Session (Friday 18.2.55)

Sammy immediately starts drawing.

First drawing: 'This door is to a place where all the people are laundry cleaners. They're nice people and they come from Israel. There's a big hospital in the back for sick people.'

J. M. – Who are these people exactly?

S. – I don't really want to tell you. I don't think I should. Oh well (with much hesitation) it's the laundry that's just by our house.

Second drawing: 'This is a path and many people come along it. There is a "Thing" which doesn't go away. It's like the other treasure. They come to see the "Thing". People will want to take it home because it's the best "Thing" in the world. Now don't say it's my penis 'cause even President Eisenhower has one. The people coming up this path are explorers. The "Thing" has no milk in it but it is full of cold hard stuff. Now who's is it? It's yours, that's all.'

I try to draw Sammy out on this fantasy. Meanwhile he puts an 'M' on the page saying that it is his idea for the next drawing. (He clearly gives me the feeling that he is thinking up ideas for drawings as a defence against going too far in probing his thoughts.)

Third drawing: 'A bunch of mimosa. There are men here in front of mirrors but they don't know that it's mirrors because all the world around is a mirror. From the distance it looks like this. (He makes a number of little pink drawings and then turns to me.) Look, Granny, the little pink things are amusements.'

J. M. – Why do you call me Granny?

    S. – (Looking embarrassed and angry.) Stop talking about it! It's none of your business! Besides she is my step-grandmother, because my mother's mother died. There now, you should be glad I've told you so much. But instead you want to know more.

Fourth drawing: 'All these people are in prison. They're bad. This first one broke a law. He went against the traffic lights four times. That one killed somebody, a boy of five. This one pushed somebody out of a window and he told big lies, too. This one here told bad tales on someone else and it wasn't even true. And this one, he conquered someone. The killer over there, he killed a boy of five. He only did it because he was afraid, just like everybody else. He was worried about something.'

Fifth drawing: 'This is a little thing which is living, and spits out water and takes in food. You know what it is? It's my behind.' (Sammy comes over and taps me lightly on the cheek because it seemed I smiled.)

Sixth drawing: 'This is a big cross with little crosses all round. It's a grave on the top of a mountain. Whose is it?'

J. M. – Well, you tell me.

    S. – Okay, it's mine. Look I'll draw my whole grave, and then I'll draw yours.

It no longer occurs to Sammy to ask me to write down what he says, but he still needs the narcissistic reassurance of having the previous day's session read back. He also dictates exactly what I am to put on each drawing. All the 'death' themes are undoubtedly stirred up by the threat of Sammy's being sent to the Special School. Today he draws our two graves side by side. All the materials related to the theme of 'fusion-in-death' has been prematurely stimulated I think, because of the spate of talk in Sammy's home about the boarding school project. Does Sammy think the Special School is 'a prison for bad people'?

76th Session (Saturday 19.2.55)

Sammy arrives today with a little clay model, carefully wrapped, which he has made at school. He makes a great mystery of this object, saying he really must not show it to me, then trying to find if there are not any special conditions which will permit him to show it, etc. etc. Finally it is brought out. It is a little sun-dried model which has been fired and painted, of a nude man, his bottom and penis clearly modelled. The man's hands are out-spread and have holes to hold candles.

> S. – See, he's quite naked. I made him for when there are visitors at home. (Sammy's mother had told me that she thought Sammy's greatest delight was to embarrass the family in front of visitors. Sammy, however, was not particularly conscious of this. His anxiety in front of others predominated.) Why do you think I made it, Dougie?
> J. M. – Perhaps it was a way of showing yourself to visitors.
> S. – You're right! I'm sure it's that!

(On the read-back of this session the following day Sammy for once disagreed, saying, 'I don't think I really said that. I wouldn't do it you know, not in front of guests'.)

There followed a long discussion of the technicalities of pottery making.

> S. – Oh boy! I'm so proud of this candlestick! Now let's draw.

144

This is a ship going away fast and carrying the people towards a thing they do not know. Here's the whole world and the ocean all around and the name of this is the Hipposidic Ocean. These people are now on an island, and the Thing seems to be following them. Now we can have many different pictures of the Thing. It keeps changing shape, and it can make a spooky sound. But it's not hurting them. Everyone is trying to see it with their magic telescopes. It is shaped a bit like a Y, and there's this circle all round it. The thing is made . . . well . . . it might be something like the way new planets come into existence. Now tell me what it is, Dougie.

Sammy taps the Thing and sings the Funeral March. He is unable to give me any associations, and in fact gets most agitated when I don't come up with an explanation. He goes over all the details again, and since it seems to me that he is still exploring his fantasies of the primal scene, I ask him to draw some more pictures of the Thing to help us to understand.

> S. – Well, here in the next drawing the Thing is in two parts and one is inside the other, and then there's another drawing and you can see that they are all broken up and now they are flashing in the sky, picking up pieces and tearing away.
>
> J. M. – Well, Sammy, I think the Thing is an interest in how new things get born, like planets, or babies. So maybe it's all about the ideas you had as a little boy about how your mother and father might make a new baby, like your little sister. Sammy's tense and agitated little face relaxes immediately.
>
> S. – Oh that could be it, oh I'm so pleased! Yes, the Thing is about my parents making love and making my sister.
>
> J. M. – And then those other two drawings of the Thing might tell us something more. I think the first one where there are two things, and you said they just want to be together and you drew them one inside the other, I think this is one idea you have about your parents in bed together, and making love and it's not frightening. But the second picture where the two things are all jagged and flashing in the sky might be another kind of idea about them, but this time a frightening one. In this idea they could be tearing and hurting and doing something dangerous to each other.

Sammy then makes one last drawing entitled 'Eyes of Dougie who sees everything.'

His anxiety over the primal scene fantasies are reminiscent of his anxieties over anal excitement; anal fantasies of child-birth are also apparent.

77th Session (Monday 21.2.55)

S. – I want to drink some milk — cow's milk.

He comes over and taps my breasts to the strains of the Funeral march.

S. – Let's see Saturday's drawing, and all those thoughts I have about my parents. Well now here's another one. Can you find a thought to it? It's a man beside a book and this man wants to know what the book is about. It's a very famous book for many things. Very thick with 1097929 pages, and a great wideness in it. So what can it be about? The pages are so big and so long. It was even longer than the man's ruler. He's a great sort of scientist. No no that. Well yeah, he likes to find things out. He writes science stories about the moon and the earth.
Now here's another one. There is a knife and a knife, and a gun and a gun.

Sammy puts a cross at the point of each knife, and then a cross at the end of the guns. He points to the end of the guns.

S. – Know what this is at the ends? It's flesh! A piece of somebody's flesh. Oh ladies! It's not mine, because mine is on me. And don't go thinking that it's yours either, Dougie, because you've got yours. It's good red juicy bloody flesh. This gun shot somebody. Nice good dark blood, and see here, it's dripping on to the table. It drips into this pot which is four inches high. And here's the blood. It comes up to three inches high. Oh ladies! How much blood there is! It's good flesh, so red it hurts the eyes. Oh, ladies, you can eat, but it's meant for animals.

Sammy draws the four bits of flesh dripping with blood, then begins to stab at the paper with the pencil, yelling ferociously. He adds two more crosses, one on either side of the ensemble.

S. – The thing I want to know, whose flesh is this? And whose knives, whose table, and whose guns? Do I know the people whose flesh got killed?

J. M. – Well there's the idea about killing people, but there's also the idea of eating their flesh too. The glass you have drawn for the blood is exactly the same as that glass of milk. When little children think of eating people, it sometimes means they want to have them right inside them. It could be a way of loving people too.

S. – Oh Dougie, it's right. Because I love you, and that's what this drawing means. It's you and the people in my family. Oh what an interesting one! Now I've got such a good idea.

(He chuckles happily to himself while he makes the next drawing. It is a complicated drawing which begins as a skeleton, with foot-prints in its wake. He adds winged creatures, and sings snatches of Beethoven all the while. The sun is added and 'God with his all-seeing eyes'. This drawing is identical with 'Dougie's All-seeing Eyes' of last week. He then sketches in a church, and prints the word 'death'.)

S. – One day a mean bad beast found this man just having fun, just eating. Then the man decided to go to sleep. He was all alone, on vacation, so he just slept out. Then he heard foot-steps. Suddenly someone gripped him from the back of his neck, gripped his gobulous flesh, and poked his heart out! That . . . man . . . died! The great thing did it! A three-toed monster. See—his head isn't very well on. Now angels come down and take the man to heaven. Here on the side is the tail of the big beast, and over there God is watching. Good on one side, evil on the other. All these people are trying to touch the crosses. Everything, to the eyes of these people has crosses over it. It's like a mirage.

Sammy seems to head off an idea of drinking up my breasts at the beginning of the session, and sings the Funeral March over them instead. I am sure he is worried about the possibility of being sent to the Special School. Is the 'famous book' all the stories he has dictated to me? Did he suspect before I did, that we might really produce a book? This would be one way of not losing our analytic work, but another is in the primitive

flesh and blood eating which follows. Some rough oedipal
justice follows in the next theme where the man (Sammy) 'is
just having fun eating' and gets his heart poked out by a
mean beast. Perhaps 'the all-seeing eyes' are to cross the ocean
to America and keep Sammy safe.

78th Session (Tuesday 22.2.55)

S. – I've been having pains in my heart, and in my inside. My
mother told me to talk to you about it. Why do you think I
have them?

J. M. – What are heart pains?

S. – Monsieur Dupont gets them all the time.

Sammy goes on to give me an intricate and detailed description of
Mr Dupont's heart pains, culled from things he had overheard, and
explanations furnished by his teacher to the children to explain her
husband's illness.

J. M. – Maybe you are trying to be Monsieur Dupont.

S. – You know last night I listened to the Seventh Symphony right
through. I sat very still and quiet, and when I heard the
Funeral March I thought of everything that happens here.

(Sammy also indicates here that his heart pains are connected
with leaving.)

First drawing. 'A boat with a flag all black. A second flag, blue
and white with a big cross on it. This is a good boat with good people
on it.'

J. M. – Who are they?

S. – People who believe in Jesus like my mother and father.

J. M. – Your mother and father are in the boat?

At this remark, Sammy immediately throws the drawing aside,
and begins to splash ink around. At one moment he looks at me as
though trying to judge my reaction, and then draws a large mouth
with enormous teeth.

J. M. – Perhaps you're afraid I will eat you because you are splashing
ink all around my room?

148

Sammy nods seriously, and goes on to another drawing which illustrates another exciting fantasy relation and is called 'What I would like to do to Dougie'. It depicts a pair of women's legs, with high heeled shoes on and an enormous hand coming from the other side of the page as though it were going under the skirts. (Fig. 3.)

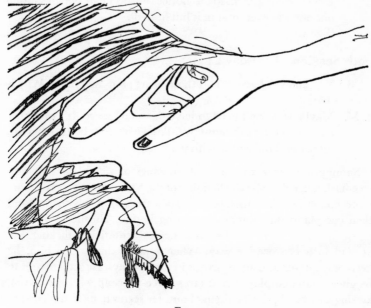

FIG. 3

S. – I'd like to put my hand up inside your skirt.
J. M. – Do you remember you had the same idea some time ago, when you were afraid I might eat your penis? I wonder if you want things between us to go on being dangerous all the time?
S. – Yes, sometimes I do. But I'm not afraid any more that you might bite off my penis. There—it's somebody's. Tell me the thought.

He has now drawn 'a penis which touches a breast'.

J. M. – Can't you tell me?

Sammy comes over and balances on the arm of my chair asking me to hold his hands and not let him fall. Meanwhile he does his level best to fall off on to the floor.

149

S. – Come on. Hold on to me tight. You said you would always protect me. Hold me Dougie, please. You know all my secrets.

Sammy wants me to hold him in France, in analysis I think. Before leaving he made a 'notice' for his chair which said no one else was ever to sit in it but himself.

79th Session (Thursday 24.2.55)

S. – You know, I haven't had those heart pains any more. Why is that?

J. M. – Maybe you don't need to have them any more. It's probably a way of telling a thought by talking with your body. After all, there's nothing wrong with your heart.

Sammy then makes a series of drawings of which the first represents damage done by the flooding of the Seine, so that there are no more houses left in Paris. He makes a series along this theme, and then complains that things are getting boring. He starts to throw plasticine around the walls, and begins tentatively flicking ink around in a provocative way. When I point this out to him, he becomes agitated and aggressive as in the old days. He screams out to be given matches, plays like a cross three-year-old with the chairs, kicking them and pushing them about. He seems to have returned to all his earlier regressive reactions to anxiety. The rest of the session he spends in playing trains, and I just let him go, feeling he may need a respite of this kind.

80th Session (Friday 25.2.55)

Sammy brings with him today a series of drawings he has already made at school with the intention of bringing them here to show me. There is the Seine almost empty of water, a women talking, some people who are moving around in a cloud, a turkey about to drink, a turkey having taken a drink and a couple of drawings of horses. Sammy spends his time explaining where he had had the ideas for his drawings. They nearly all include reference to his mother, no matter where the explanations begin. I draw Sammy's attention to this and ask him if he feels that it was easier to do these drawings outside of analysis, especially those which had to do with his mother, rather than to talk about it here with me. I made no further notes on the session except to say that it was calm and defensive. On the way to join his mother, Sammy exclaimed, 'Oh, you've got new shoes on.' To her embarrassment he sits down to feel her feet in the new shoes. She remarks to me that Sammy is always fascinated by her shoes, and loves to pick her foot up and place it down rhythmically, saying she is like a little horse.

> S.–(To me.) Perhaps this has something to do with my horse drawings too?

(Faced with threatened separation, Sammy is already detaching himself from analysis by interpreting his own drawing.)

81st Session (Saturday 26.2.55)

Sammy arrives covered in iodine to disinfect a minute scratch. He displays the scratch and the precautionary treatment, with much squeaking and pleasure.

> S.–Guess what I made at Ginette's place . . . clay models . . . oooh. . . . If I tell you about it you'll be mad. Oooooh. I made it because it's something to worry about. I shouldna' done it. It's too big. You're gonna get oh so mad, so good and mad!
>
> J. M.–It sounds as though you hope I will.
>
> S.–No. If you got really mad . . . well, there's the trouble. You see, I made it and it's so big. I made Ginette's . . . oooh . . . oooh . . . but it's her really. A clay portrait of her. But that's not the trouble. Oooooh you're going to get as mad as can be. Sakes alive. I made *me* too. But me and her *together* and here's the trouble—me and her are both *naked*! And I even made her bosoms!
>
> J. M.–The way you talk about it, it's as though you're afraid I'm going to be jealous.

I link this interpretation up with other things we have talked about recently concerning Sammy's own feelings of jealousy, and his projection of these on to me or others: his fear that his mother would be jealous of his attachment to me, his fierce jealousy of other patients, whether child or adult, and the notice for his chair. I do not

151

recall exactly where this material appeared in the sessions, since I now only make rough notes after Sammy's sessions. But the jealousy themes have run through the sessions of the last few weeks like a constant thread.

> S. – May I bring these little drawings over to you so you can see them close up?

I allow this, and it turns out to be a ruse so that Sammy may attempt to push his hands up under my skirts. I forbid this, but suggest that he draws what he wants to do. He draws again two legs under a skirt with an enormous hand which moves towards them.

> S. – Guess what! That's me. And it looks as though you're going to take something away from me at the same time. Now how could that be possible?

He follows this with 'a tiny vine with bits of joyfulness all round it. And leaves are flying through the air. We know what *that* means' (a reference to the anal animal games).

> J. M. – Troubles coming? When you think of things we could take from one another, you are worried about all those penis-bosom ideas. And it makes you want to go back to the time of worrying about the fart-fart too.
> S. – Yes. But I can make *signs* now instead. Here is a sign that stands for good. It is a cross drawn over a circle, and the cross by itself means bad.

82nd Session (Monday 28.2.55)

Sammy arrives rather late on this occasion, and spends the greater part of the session showing me how competent he is at long division. From time to time he asks for my help.

> J. M. – Perhaps you feel safer here with me as a teacher than as an analyst today?
> S. – But I *want* to do this.
> J. M. – I'm sure it's interesting and that you are learning lots of new things at school, but perhaps also there is something you would rather not talk to me about today.

S. – Oh yeah. I must have my analysis. No one has sat in my chair
   I hope? Promise?

He begins to draw with his face all contorted in anger, then he
seems to relax and begins to hum a tune.

S. – Now this is a man looking very angry, out of a window.
   Someone he knows has been killed, over there where you see
   the cross. Someone killed him, at five after two. You know I
   went to a new place for school today, and there was a new
   lady to look after us too. I don't know her name. Oh and
   I must tell you that I've got heart pains and pains down
   there. (He points to his genitals.) And let's see, there's a third
   one. Wait a bit, ooh yes, it's on my right side, an appendix
   ache.

He goes on to recount incidents from 'Tom Sawyer' with particular
interest in the passage where the boys hide the fact that they want to
vomit, and where everybody believes them to be dead.

S. – I don't feel well. I feel like vomiting a bit.

The next day Sammy did not come. His mother phoned to say he
was ill.

83rd Session (Thursday 3.3.55)

Sammy brings a bunch of drawings done at school to which Mme
Dupont, his teacher, had given 'thoughts' at Sammy's request.

S. – I like her thoughts better than yours. They're much prettier.
   And I've a right to think whatever I want to!
J. M. – You feel you have to protect yourself against me?

One of the drawings is of a man sitting on top of a house, and
beside him a large cross. Sammy has written Mme Dupont's interpretation around the drawing, to the effect that the drawing is about
God who watches over everybody and especially loves Sammy. After
explaining this thought to me, Sammy searches out a needle and
starts to plunge it into his finger.

S. – I brought this along so I could see if my blood is good or bad.

153

He then asks me to look at last time's session notes, which are no longer dictated but are rough notes jotted down later. He is particularly interested in talking about Tom Sawyer's seeming death, and mimes death himself.

J. M. – You seem to be very interested in ideas about death, Sammy. Perhaps when you think about yourself being dead, it is a way of being able to feel close to other people?

S. – You know, I often think about it, and I imagine everyone around me all weeping and crying and sitting around my grave, and that makes me feel good.

Sammy's depressive themes are becoming constant. There is much talk about the Special School and I think he is trying different fantasy means of detaching himself from his analysis.

84th Session (Friday 4.3.55)

Sammy announces on arrival that he has something very special to show me. He explains, after much mystery, that it is a photo of Butch. I have already learnt from Sammy's parents that Butch is an American Negro boy of 12 whom Sammy met at a summer camp. The parents describe Butch as a popular boy, non-neurotic, well developed for his age and very intelligent. Sammy tells me that Butch is only one of his many boy friends. He is most sorry for me because I could never possibly have as many friends as he. He just hasn't talked of all these friends up till now because there were so many other things to say, etc. etc. This long, exaggerated story gives me a glimpse of Sammy's awareness of his acute loneliness, and how much he would like to have friends like other people. He hesitates a long time yet before deciding to show me Butch's photo.

J. M. – You seem to be afraid to show me Butch's photo.
S. – Oh yes! He's my friend. You can't have him!
J. M. – Are you afraid I shall want to take him away from you? Just the way you're afraid I want to take so many good things from you?
S. – Yes you would. But you can't! What would you say if Butch was coming up the road and you saw me run forward to hug him?

J. M. – You seem to think I would be jealous and want to keep him all to myself.

    S. – Oh yes, you'd be very jealous, and very mad.

Sammy makes great game of showing the photo, covering it up, slowly revealing certain portions of it, asking me to guess all kinds of factual data about Butch's physical appearance and so on.

    S. – And you know Butch used to kiss me. Over and over he would. You see he *really* liked me.

J. M. – You mean he liked you better than I do?

    S. – Yes. You wouldn't ever do that.

Sammy then wants to write a letter to Butch, but this idea presents endless moral difficulties to him. He asks reassurance that it is in order to write to Butch in my house. He wants to know if anyone else has ever done such a thing in an analytic session.

J. M. – You seem to feel there is something wrong or bad about writing to your friend.

    S. – Well, I'm not sure if it's done. Oh I suppose it's alright.

He then passes the rest of the session in writing this letter. It is edited and re-edited, and finally achieved. The letter is colourless, meagre, and mostly limited to weather conversation and other banal remarks. Nevertheless, Sammy is pleased with it, largely I think because he has managed to write something without the slightest emotional tone to it. His pleasure in showing me that he has now learned to write is also marked, and I am myself astonished at his progress.

> Precipitated by the threatened departure, Sammy brings me this 'homosexual' love for his friend and dares me to take it away. He has also made so much progress in his own feeling of separateness and identity that he now turns to Butch, hoping to gain through him a valuable masculine identification, but he is frightened as always, by the erotisation of his needs.

85th Session (Saturday 5.3.55)

Sammy arrives early and in an agitated frame of mind. After being shown to the waiting-room by Hélène, he comes charging into the consulting-room (the first time he has ever done this), interrupts a session with an adult patient and goes out in a state of considerable embarrassment. He has brought a framed picture that he has made himself, to show me. It was painted for a friend of the family whom Sammy considers to be a very good friend of his.[1]

From talking about this man he passes to discussing Butch. 'You won't get him from me,' he cries. He then asks to have the box of paints, for the first time since the beginning of his analysis.

He is very annoyed to find that the box has already been used and that it is not the same box he had some months ago. He demands a new box, and is truly distraught when I tell him there is no other. He criticises the colours in the box, finding them unsuited to the painting he has in mind, makes brownish marks on the paper, and tries to put paint on me. Asks with great irritation if other children use this paintbox and finally begins to draw on the carpet.

J. M. – You are angry with me because I see other patients besides you, Sammy. And especially today because you came in and saw me with a man. Perhaps you feel jealous of the others.

S. – Well, never mind!! But I've a secret to tell. Oh but you won't do it! It's no use!

He makes a great pantomime over this secret, pretending to be terrified to tell it, but finally gets it out. He wants to listen to music with me here one day, on my gramophone.

He follows this request with many questions about whether such a thing is done, whether any other patient would think of making such a request and so on. He obviously feels extremely guilty about all his music fantasies.

J. M. – You think it might be a bad thing to listen to music here with me?

S. – I don't know. It might be dangerous. Oh oh oh, I wish I knew if I could. Perhaps we could do it after the Easter holidays. You know *you* might like it Dougie. I know, you just tell me when you would like to hear some music with me, and then we'll have it. You just let me know Dougie!

J. M. – You seem to want me to take the responsibility. I wonder why you're afraid to ask yourself.

[1] Mrs Y told me that the man in question found Sammy's attentions most embarrassing. Sammy would ask him if he could look at the hair on his chest and legs, and would slide his hands under the man's shirt and make suggestive remarks.

S. – I don't think it's what we ought to be doing, and my mother
mightn't like it either.

J. M. – You're afraid your mother might get angry about the things
we do together here?

S. – Yes!! Well, I don't know. She likes me to listen to music at
home. Music is very good for me. You know it's good for the
insides.

Sammy squirms around in his chair, squeaking and squealing at
the thought of listening to music here. He asks endless questions.
Shall it be my music or his? What would I say if he played the
Beethoven Seventh? And what would happen when we came to the
Funeral March?

S. – There's something that puzzles me. I don't any longer want
to listen to the Fifth Symphony and it used to be my favourite.
Why would that be?

J. M. – Might it be because of all the fart-fart stories and all the other
ideas we talked about in connection with that music?

S. – (Nodding vigorously.) Oh yes, that's it. But then everyone
gets tired of listening to a symphony when they listen to it too
often. That's quite natural.

86th Session (Monday 7.3.55)

S. – Here's a drawing of the sun and the moon together. Now
guess the right meaning.

J. M. – Perhaps there are things in your mind you would like me to
guess at rather than tell me yourself?

S. – Ah, you're afraid of something happening to you if you guess.
No, no, I have it or at least part of it, you're afraid I will be
angry if you guess right.

J. M. – I guess you would like to psychoanalyse me, Sammy.

Later on he wonders if I show his paintings to others who come
here. He wants to know what I would do if I found another boy
looking at his pictures, and I tell him that I think he is jealous of what
he imagines others do here with me.

S. – Well the trouble is you don't like me.

J. M. – Perhaps you feel safe believing that.

S. – Oh, I know it by the way you act.

157

He does not elaborate on this idea, but goes on to finish his painting and comments that he paints 'better' than when he first came to see me. In explanation of this he says, 'You see in this drawing, although that tree on the left is nearly dead, those to the right are good and living'. (He can now conceive of the other ways out than death.)

87th Session (Tuesday 8.3.55)

S. – Two grown-ups and a young man of 12 or 13 live here. There is a budding tree and two lively ones. Now tell me what the other children do who come to see you.

J. M. – What do you think the others do here?

S. – Do they show you their behinds? I'll never take my pants down for you! Do the others worry about what the others do?

Sammy wants me to tell him exactly what he must paint today. I tell him that he seems to want me to control what he does so as to make it safe, or perhaps to be sure to do the same things as the other children.

S. – Yeah, I know — but tell me all the same. I say, Dougie, what would you say if I smeared you all over with brown paint?

J. M. – That it was some sort of lavatory game you wanted to play with me.

S. – Well, if it were another colour?

J. M. – It wouldn't make any difference to my feeling about it.

S. – I'm going to paint what I see when I listen to the Seventh Symphony!

(He paints for some time singing snatches of Beethoven all the while. More interest in colour and movement than in form. Squeezes white paint directly on to the paper singing the Funeral March and smiling at me, then paints in some roses saying they look just the way he sees them in the Symphony. He is very pleased with his painting.)

88th Session (Thursday 10.3.55)

Sammy talks about a coming visit to Le Havre which he will make in the company of his father.

S. – I can hardly wait. I'm so glad you're not coming. You'll be
here all alone in your little dump. (Hums the Funeral March
over the paints, saying he does not want to paint today.) Oh,
I'm so glad *you're* not coming to Le Havre! You might spoil it
all. Will you miss me while I'm away? Oh no, you won't—
not you! Now this drawing is a stone building which hangs so
high in the sky. I thought of nothing when I wrote the
numbers on it, but now I remember I have a camera film
which is marked 127. No thought? What a shame.

He scribbles gaily, grinning, making grimaces, bizarre tongue
movements and jerky movements of his head. He takes up again the
current question about the other patients and deduces answers for
himself.

S. – Any girls come here? I wonder what could be wrong with
them. What's the matter with grown-ups who come to see
you? Did nobody ever have troubles like mine?
J. M. – What troubles are you thinking of, Sammy?
S. – It's a pretty damn shame if you don't know my troubles by
now! What are my troubles? All the children that I don't play
well enough with. Oh, I wish you'd tell me if there's anyone
else like me. If I were the only one with troubles like me I
wouldn't like it. Well? I guess there isn't anyone else because
you don't say so. Oh, I can't be the *only* one! I have an idea, I
want to draw something but it's so babyish. It's a real trouble
but I won't tell it to you because all your patients will be told
and they will make a big shame of me. Oh, it's so babyish!
And I like it. It's not easy to talk about. . . . Like the fart-fart.
More babyish. I wonder what you'd say if you knew. I want
to know thoughts to this when I tell you. Do you have any
new patients coming?

To the majority of these questions I give no answer or ask why it
interests him.

S. – Kid—the next time you ask why I would like to know something you'll be slapped in the face, so you'll know you've done
wrong not to tell me!
J. M. – It seems you want to be the boss and ask all the questions and
keep everything under control.

159

S. – Oh, I like that idea—yeah! That's right. You can just go right on talking.

J. M. – There you go again!

S. – What do you call kings who get like that? You know people who say things like 'Go get water so the babies may drink'. Oh yes, you can call me Nebuchadnezzah. Oh, I feel good now. Mr Bossy King. When you talk to me just call 'Listen, Oh King'. I wonder if others make drawings and hide them. I know, will you draw me? I'll pose.

Sammy poses and becomes so insistent and so truly enraged when I do not start immediately to draw him that I give in. My efforts are met with trenchant criticism.

S. – Well, never mind, just put some little things coming out of my head will you? If I had a portrait of you it will have those. Any thought to this? Old horn-headed lady!

J. M. – You seem to ge giving me a sort of penis once again.

S. – Oh, I'm glad I'm bigger and better than you. Oh my fuckin's, am I glad!

The homosexual protection through a paternal object is now expressed in the reality situation of Sammy's trip with his father. As at the beginning of treatment, this allows Sammy to form a secondary identification with his father but on more developed and classical oedipal lines. This situation is, in any case, infinitely more reassuring to him than that with his analyst. His jubilation when he imagines himself as king of the realm is, no doubt, more a mockery than real, since he cannot reign long without encountering frustration from the mother. At the very most, he can issue orders in her place to fetch and carry water 'for the babies to drink'. He is also concerned about who might take his place—another patient or a new baby.

89th Session (Friday 11.3.55)

Sammy says he can hardly wait for tomorrow to leave with his father. He sits down rapidly and clumsily, hitting his foot on the side of the chair.

S. – (Wailing.) Ow! I broke a bone. King Sammy is now on his throne! (He does a drawing.) This is my boat in case you ever become my enemy. It has all my ladies aboard. All ready to fight if ever need be. I know it couldn't really. Now here are two countries, yours and mine, and there's the secret I talked about. Oh my, oh my! (He carries on for some time lamenting his inability to tell me the secret.) Oh dear, not many boys of my age still like looking at them. It's babyish! I didn't tell you yesterday. I wonder if I will today. Now don't say a word when you see what it is. Be as silent as if you were in a church.

He draws, singing the Funeral March, covering the drawing with his hand. Then makes a cover sheet to place over it, and a sheet over the cover sheet. The whole thing is then covered with crosses and passed to me. Inside is a drawing of a train.

J. M. – Why is it so difficult to tell, Sammy?

S. – The trouble is that I want to play with my ruler and pretend it's a train. I like doing it but I don't want to think that it's *not bad*. I know it must be bad. How can I stop it? Oh my, what will happen to me? If I just don't do it for a few nights perhaps it'll be alright. I keep thinking to myself it's no good, the only way to get out of the habit is not to do it.

J. M. – I think we'll get to understand it quite well and you won't have to feel bad about it.

> To understand why Sammy finds playing with trains so guilt-making, we must take into account:
> (*a*) that he is to set out the following day with his father;
> (*b*) that any symbolic activity is for him highly cathected, despite the struggle he wages against such cathexis;
> (*c*) that playing with trains must arouse in him, as it frequently does in younger children, omnipotent masturbatory fantasies.
>
> In contradiction to normal children, the intense guilt associated with symbolic activity makes play almost impossible for Sammy.

90th Session (Monday 14.3.55)

Sammy gives a minutely detailed account of his trip to Le Havre and the visit, *en route*, to Rouen where they spent two hours 'because of Joan of Arc'. Amongst other things, he wanted to cross himself in the Cathedral at Rouen but he was afraid his father would not approve of this. He slept in the same room as his father at the hotel and was allowed the choice of beds. These seemed to be the salient features of his week-end. He asks many questions about my activities while he was away and what I had done at his missed session on Saturday, and what I had done with other patients.

> S. – I had a dream last night that you were pregnant. I'm so glad it's not true.
> J. M. – Perhaps you were afraid I might do as your mother did and make a baby sister, and I think it's the same reason which makes you ask so many questions about the other patients today.
> S. – I don't care about my sister. You'll never guess what happened today.

Sammy tries to tell me but is too anxious to get the words out. He finally writes a note to me saying that today a priest came to school. A most dreadful experience: he will never go back if that happens again. He was intensely afraid. 'There is nothing so bad as a bad priest' and he begins to mime the way in which a bad priest behaves. Wearing a diabolical expression he moves towards his empty chair and makes threatening gestures around it. 'But there can be good priests too.' He mimes the good priest whose gestures are equally terrifying. The good priest act consists of Sammy sobbing, crying and finally hiding behind the curtain and screaming. After a moment he emerges and asks if I would mind playing the role of a priest. I ask what I am supposed to do and am told that I must 'frown and frown'. I am to stand up and make these frowns towards my own chair. I do this while Sammy screams, 'Oh, I hope it doesn't come to me, I hope it doesn't come to me!' in a tone of excited terror. Meanwhile he encourages me by every means to come towards his chair and to make him afraid.

J. M. – What is it that makes you afraid?

Sammy suddenly picks up a sheet of paper and makes a drawing: a face with two breasts attached to it. On one of the breasts is written 'very good milk in it' and on the other he writes 'bad, bad milk'. Around the breasts he draws a star of David and a cross and adds a second cross to the breast with bad milk in it. While doing so he tells me he is Jewish and that I am Catholic. He then asks for a glass of milk, and meanwhile adds the names 'Sammette' 'Dougette' to the drawing.

J. M. – You want me to give you milk but you're also afraid that it'll be bad.

Sammy impatiently pushes the bell to summon Hélène who brings him a glass of milk which he drinks immediately. He writes at the top of the page 'Very bad milk' and immediately follows this by saying 'Mmmmmmm that was good'. On a second page he draws a heart with many hearts inside it.

S. – Guess whose?

He then draws the cathedral of Rouen and puts a cross on the house of Joan of Arc 'because something bad happened to her'. He recounts that while in the Cathedral he had bent down simply to fix his shoe and had asked his father if the others would think he was praying, and that his father had found this very funny. He then draws a map of France, England and New York. France is marked 'sad', England is covered with a cross, and New York is smiling.

After the session, Mrs Y tells me she has had another letter from the Director of the Special School who will interview Sammy in Paris next month.

> The importance of Sammy's trip with his father is enhanced by his need for a 'homosexual' refuge, but this in turn is felt to be dangerous. This is the reversal of the oedipal drive manifest in the dream where Sammy sees his analyst-mother as pregnant (and thus proves that he did not steal father for himself away from mother).
>
> The priest's visit allows Sammy to analyse his relationship with an ambiguous figure which is both male and female, good and bad like the breasts. Sammy feels the transference situation to be as ambiguous and dangerous as that which he has just experienced with the priest. The analyst is a good mother and a good breast, a bad mother and a bad breast.

91st Session (Tuesday 15.3.55)

Sammy spends most of the session talking of the Special School. First, he is afraid of leaving me and not being able to go on with his

163

analysis; second, he feels he will miss his school teachers and his small school class a great deal; third, he is afraid there will be a large number of children in the new school; fourth, he is afraid of separating from his parents.

He asks many questions, such as, 'What sort of character do you think the Director has?', 'Is he like Dr Lebovici whom I saw once?', 'Do you think he has a wife?', 'Are the other children there dumb and stupid? I'm afraid there will be children who can't talk properly', 'Perhaps the food is not good', 'Maybe there are some children at this school who don't want to talk about their troubles. Those children won't get better.' 'But', he adds philosophically, 'I don't think that's my particular problem.'

> S. – Dougie, could you promise me that when I leave that school I will really have no further troubles.
>
> J. M. – The school is there to help people with troubles.
>
> S. – But I'm so full of troubles it might take a long time. Besides, I don't want to go there. My parents said if I tried to behave better at home and be my age, I could go to regular school and then I'd be able to stay in Paris. Oh I'll try, I'll try. I'll do everything I can to please them. Even if I have to go to a boarding school in Paris. I wish that American school didn't exist.

Pathetically distressed, and knowing that I am to see his parents the next day, Sammy pleads with me to tell them all these things.

> He feels I could protect him but that I am handing him over to the man instead. I feel it is very important for Sammy to continue with his analysis and tell his parents this when I see them later that evening. In any case no decision can be made before the Director has seen Sammy.

92nd Session (Thursday 17.3.55)

Sammy talks about the mi-carême hats being made at school for Lent.

> S. – But there's a trouble with mine. The fringe is made of toilet paper—Oooh!

164

Even this exciting detail does not help keep Sammy's mind off the school in America. He asks many questions which I am unable to answer.

S. – I wish my parents would ask me instead of just going along with their own thoughts. Why can't *you* do something, Dougie?

During this conversation Sammy wiggles around in his chair obviously wanting to urinate, but makes a great scene over it as though it were something very guilty, much in the manner of his pantomime when he asks for milk.

J. M. – Why is it so troubling to want to go to the lavatory? What might happen?

S. – Your breasts might come after me and attack my penis if I tell you what I'm thinking.

Sammy does not divulge what these thoughts might be and asks me to guess. He continues with many questions about what other children do here and returns again to his sadness at possibly having to leave. He draws 'A huge thing on a mountain'. This Thing has great feet and large arms with big sleeves. In front of it there is a cross with a 'cloth draped behind it, in corduroy velvet'. (I am wearing a corduroy velvet skirt.)

S. – The head behind the mountain, we don't know if it's good or bad. But there's a skeleton at the side here. Perhaps this person killed that man whose skeleton we can see. It might be God, we don't know.

J. M. – I think this frightening person might be an idea that you have of me. After all you said a short while ago that I might attack your penis and sometimes you have had the idea that God was part of me—besides I am wearing a corduroy skirt. So I guess you still see me as a very dangerous and very powerful, Sammy.

S. – Hmmmmmm—yes that's true.

He goes on to make a drawing of a ship to which he tells a confused story. It is followed by several other sketchy drawings which I can make nothing of. He places a cover sheet over all the day's drawing and writes on it:

'Sammy
My Hart'

165

Sammy's ambivalence is marked throughout the session: I fail to protect him from being sent away, I menace him with castration, my breasts pursuing his penis, and I contain the 'huge thing' hidden by my skirt and placed under the sign of the cross.

93rd Session (Friday 18.3.55)

S.–Oh Dougie, you must do something about that school in America. My parents say they're doing it for my happiness. But it doesn't make me at all happy to leave here. I don't understand what they're talking about.

Sammy makes five drawings.

First drawing: 'A chimney-place with three objects on it. A cup in which something is burning, a lid and a third object which nobody knows anything about.' (This drawing resembles strikingly the 'oedipal situation' depicted at his very first session.)

Second drawing: 'A cross.' As soon as this drawing is finished, Sammy rushes around to my side of the table and starts pushing his hand up under my skirt. However, he returns peacefully to his chair when I ask him to do so. Such sexual sallies always precipitate punitive thoughts in Sammy. He now draws 'Death coming from over the Hill'. On one side 'three crosses with three fires' and 'some bad stuff on the other side'. I ask him what this might mean and he says 'perhaps a person with no head or someone with a tail'.

J. M.–Perhaps it's someone who seems dangerous as I seemed to you yesterday. When I don't protect you, you feel as though you could lose your head or your tail.

Fourth drawing: 'Four good men in a war.'

S.–Bad men start the war because the good ones have things the bad ones have not. The first man is getting whipped, you can see the blood running. The second is nearly dead with a knife stuck in him, the third is already dead and the fourth has just been killed with a hammer in his back. At the side a chief of the camp is seeing to it that everything goes well. (Fig. 4.)

J. M.–Perhaps you are still wanting to get out all the fear you have about me wanting to take away the good things *you* have.

166

S. – Ah yes, my penis.

J. M. – Yes, and perhaps other things too. These could be stories of dangers you imagine might happen to you if you spend too much time with me. Perhaps you feel the need of a man like the chief of a camp to protect you really.

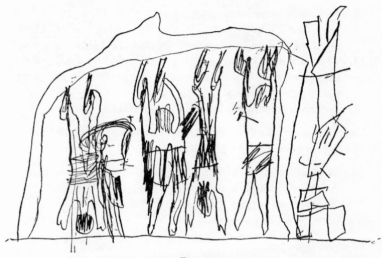

Fig. 4

At this moment the door bell rings, 'Ah there's my mother' says Sammy. He rapidly does a fifth drawing, 'Two vultures and a little baby one in between them.'

J. M. – Perhaps these vultures are your mother and me who you feel might eat you all up, and maybe the little baby is the way you feel when you would like to eat us all up?

This interpretation of Sammy's oral-sadistic imagery pleases him. He grins and runs out.

> I think he also feels that his mother and I are the bad ones who are going to let him be sent away; this fits his pregenital image of mother-figures.

94th Session (Saturday 19.3.55)

On this session I only noted that Sammy wanted to listen to music and spent the whole time trying to find the courage to play a record.

He finally did so and before going out whispered, 'I was afraid you would do something to me'.

95th Session (Monday 21.3.55)

S. – My mother says I may not have to go to that school until next year. But I don't want to go at all!! Today I'm not afraid anything will happen or anything. So can I listen to music?

J. M. – There seems to be a frightening idea behind the music all the same. You once told me that music was made to be eaten and put in your insides.

S. – But that's true. Music is good for your insides.

He looks through a pile of records and puts one on. (The Beethoven Violin Concerto in D Major.) We listen for about half a minute.

S. – Don't look so serious like you're just going to pay your income tax! Music's for pleasure—what's the matter with you.

After another two or three minutes' listening:

S. – Oooh, Ginette's bottom, I love to hit it, she's so round and plump. Just like meat!

(Sammy is still little reassured about the rightness of listening to music here. Among its many pregenital connotations it also represents reciprocal anal activity. He asks if other children listen to music, and what people would think of such children. Although he accepts that music represents a pleasure which is thought of as being bad, he is unable to go very much further with this.)

S. – But I think I'm alright. I never have heart pains now. But I still have a trouble. I'm still playing trains—why can't you help me with this? I want to think that it's not a bad thing to play trains. Oh that school in America will be great. The counsellors there are all very kind. They answer all your questions. Oh boy, I'm so pleased to be going there! Tell me, Dougie, do you ever look at yourself in the mirror? Do you look from top to bottom. Do you look at your behind? Why don't you tell me what I want to know? You don't love anything but your bottom. Your big smelly bottom that's always dirty and that you never wipe! (i.e. Sammy is not interested in the anal-erotic game, only Dougie.)

J. M. – Perhaps you are telling me about some things you like doing.

    S. – Tell me, how many pieces of paper do you use?

J. M. – And you?

    S. – That's none of your business!

This conversation lasts throughout the whole playing of the record to which Sammy listens only at odd moments. The music finishes just at the end of the session.

96th Session (Tuesday 22.3.55)

No mention of music today. Sammy is very excited because I am wearing a short-sleeved pullover. He tells me that in New York everyone goes naked when it gets warm. He draws 'what I hope you will look like in the summer' in which I am dressed in shorts with a low-cut blouse. His second drawing is 'Mother and Son in New York'. (Fig. 5.)

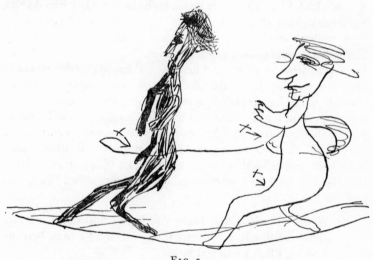

Fig. 5

    S. – Her breasts want to bite off his penis. Is there any thought behind that?

J. M. – Well, it sounds as though you think mothers are pretty dangerous for their sons.

    S. – Oh boy, yes!

The third drawing shows all the people in New York swimming in the Hudson river.

Sammy then starts to look through the folder of his drawings and begins to remember some of his earlier sessions.

> S. – I can't think why I used to feel so bored in the beginning when I came here. Perhaps it was because I didn't know you so well, and didn't know what things I was allowed to say.

Sammy's manner during this session indicated that he is coping quite differently with the anxiety aroused by pre-genital fantasy. Here he proffers a pre-genital defence (breast biting penis) against oedipal anxiety and genital affect.

97th Session (Thursday 24.3.55)

In a state of high elation Sammy talks the whole fifty minutes almost without pause. His main topics are that (i) he had an exciting day in which I had absolutely no part; (ii) he has a boy friend and is highly delighted about this. He adds that no doubt I have patients who couldn't even make a boy friend, and whose troubles are increasing instead of disappearing like his. (iii) He knows now that he is going to grow up strong and healthy and happy. (iv) At school he now does exciting things like dividing with two numbers. There are also fish swimming around amongst grass in a bowl at school and it is very important that I realise that these are his things, and I have no part in them. A little later he announces his intention of writing to his New York therapist because, unlike me, she will immediately write back and tell him all about the troubles of her other patients. He talks of a song he learned at a holiday camp, called 'You, you, you'.

> S. – When I'm older and know you better and can have love affairs with you, I will sing it to you. If I've been here six months, I'll sing it to you now.

He counts up, finds it to be six months, and writes down a few words.

> S. – This is partly true what this love song says. No, it's all true, it's really what I believe. Read it slowly then say something.

J. M. – You know you feel so full of good things today, and you need to show me that you could get along without me. But perhaps at the same time you're afraid I'll be cross because of all this—so you reassure me by telling me how much you love me.

98th Session (Friday 25.3.55)

S. – Dougie, I've thought about it. I *really* love you. Now I'm going to draw a heart with a dagger in it. This dagger has some poison in it, and the drawing stands for love.

He continues to talk about his love for me, and at the same time hits me several times on the arms. I point out to him that while talking about loving he seems at the same time to be attacking me.

S. – Yes, why so I do that? I don't understand because it's true all about my heart and my loving you.

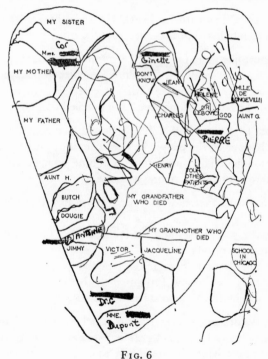

Fig. 6

171

J. M. – Perhaps it's a hitting way of loving me Sammy, as if you still aren't sure that loving me is safe. (Sammy laughs delightedly.)

S. – Yes, it really is like that.

He begins to draw a picture of his heart and all the people who are in it. The heart is divided into various small boxes 'all the same size'. Into it he places his mother, his father, his sister, his friend Butch, himself, and me; then stands back to admire it. He is suddenly distressed to find that there are so few people in his heart. (Fig. 6.)

S. – My heart is all in bits like that because I don't know some-times just how it is really. Perhaps there could be other people in it. But it means I'm not sure if I like them or not. (Sammy then adds sundry relatives.)

S. – Just look at these people all around. My, it makes me feel nice and safe.

99th Session (Saturday 26.3.55)

Sammy continues with his heart. He adds the names of certain children and includes a little corner 'for your other patients'.

S. – I must like them because I keep thinking about them, but it's only a very small bit. (He finally decides to put God into his heart in a space the size of that reserved for my patients.)

S. – Now I must make one for all the people I don't like.

He cannot decide whether he needs another heart for those or what will happen to the people he does like, if he puts those he does not like into it too. This question irritates him to such a point that he decides there is something wrong with me.

S. – What's the matter with you, you are in a bad mood aren't you?

J. M. – Maybe you're feeling a bit cross because you cannot decide about your heart?

S. – Not me, I never get angry with anybody, but I can see you're not very well today. I'm going to give you a prescription to get you better. You must listen to music.

He then writes out a prescription which says that I must take music regularly until I am better. He gives various suggestions as to the kind of music which is most likely to cure me (and my internal objects, or rather the conflict among them which he has projected on to me, along with his broken heart).

100th Session (Monday 28.3.55)

Aimless scribbles and snatches of 'this little Piggy went to Market'. At one moment he says' there are those who achieve it and some who miss it'. He again sings the nursery song followed by several others. I asked him whether what some achieve and others miss is having nursery songs sung to them such as his mother does with his baby sister.

S.–Ah, that gives me an idea for a drawing. Here's a mountain and up on its summit are all the things that people ever wanted. Down at the bottom are people trying to get there. You and I are there too. There's a secret way up to the top. The people are trying hundreds of routes, but they always miss.

J. M.–I wonder what the things are that are up on top?

S.–Don't you know? I don't either, but I thought you would.

J. M.–Well, I suppose it's something that you must have always wanted, for yourself?

S.–Yes—breasts. (He suddenly looks most embarrassed.) Oh well, I don't know why I said that—oh let's get on.

J. M.–Did you want to have breasts?

S.–Will I have them one day? No, I won't, I know I won't, but I just want to touch them—my wife's.

Sammy continues with his drawing, the people continue to try to climb the mountain, but they never arrive. 'They never found that you had to climb over the wall,' Sammy explains. 'They thought it was something they weren't allowed to do. There was even a little notice on the wall "Go On", and they were *so* near.'

Underneath his design Sammy writes 'God's Heaven', and 'Breast'.

S.–Tell me, if there is a thought behind this. What is it?

J. M.–Maybe there's a thought that you would like to become a baby again.

S.–In heaven it'll come true and everyone will have all they have ever wanted. What would you have said if the people *did* get over the wall?

173

(Sammy symbolises heaven as a return to the breast, but characteristically feels this good thing is outside and not integrated within him.)

101st Session (Tuesday 29.3.55)

No notes were taken of this session, but Sammy spent the whole time drawing mazes and line drawings with no apparent meaning. The first maze is labelled 'You'; the third has a vaguely human shape; it gives the impression of a body filled with intestines. The final drawing is entirely scribble with black and red pencil and labelled 'The End'. Perhaps the journey 'to the top of the mountain' was Sammy's picture of the analysis and he feels now that if I am to abandon him everything is a maze and a muddle. Nothing straight inside. On top of the 'Special School' threat I have also announced the forthcoming Easter break.

102nd Session (Thursday 31.3.55)

Sammy brings two dreams. 'My father was throwing me up into the air, and then it was you who was doing it. At first I was frightened, but then I found that my head went right through the roof without any trouble. In the other dream, I was with Butch, and we were rubbing our faces together. I think I dreamt about Butch because he didn't reply to my letter. Tell me what the dream about my father and you means.'

J. M. – Perhaps it means that you would like your father and me to do all sorts of exciting things to you, but at the same time they are things which seem frightening. What do you think about it?

S. – I would rather talk about Butch. Butch liked me an awful lot. Once I put my hand on his face and he put his arms around me and kissed me. He did, he did! And don't go thinking it was *my* idea. It was Butch who started it. I was really very cross with him. And then my mother said it had to stop, but it was Butch did all that. Oh, that Butch he makes me mad!

J. M. – What do you think it was that bothered you so much?

S. – Well, you can't do it—it's against the custom.

174

J. M. – Perhaps it bothered you too because you say that Butch did all these things and you just let yourself be kissed as if you felt you were being a bit like a girl?

S. – Oh no, because then Butch would not like me. He's like me, he only wants to kiss boys.

Sammy then constructs a number of imaginary situations in which I would meet Butch, and they all seem to end with my forbidding Butch to be so friendly with Sammy.

J. M. – You seem to feel that I will take Butch away from you as you say your mother did when she told you to stop the kissing. Perhaps that's why you wanted me to be more like your father than your mother in the dream?

103rd Session (Friday 1.4.55)

As Sammy rushes into the room he announces that he doesn't need me any more. He now has friends who love him, and to support this contention he shows me a drawing done by his friend Pierre at school. Sammy starts off with the intention of doing some drawing himself, but spends almost the entire session in seductive gestures towards me, putting his arms around me, trying to kiss me, and asking me to kiss him. When I ask him why he does not talk about it, instead of jumping on to my chair all the time, he looks very hurt.

S. – Oh Dougie, come on. Let's have a real love affair, Oh I feel it in my heart that you don't really love me. Give me a kiss! See how you are? I suppose you only see me for the money my mother pays you!

Sammy then writes a series of love messages. 'I love you, I love you so much, even when I'm hitting you and saying bad things to you. I don't know what my mother would think of you.'

J. M. – Perhaps you're wanting to love me in the way you want to love your mother?

S. – I can see you don't love me, and I wasn't hitting or anything. I was so gentle and loving and look how you are.

During Sammy's love-making games he has interspersed many questions regarding his relationship with Butch. Is it bad to kiss a

175

boy? Is it good to go against the custom? etc. Then he draws two heads in profile labelled 'You' and 'Me'. He finally does a full-page drawing of a heart divided into many small pieces and labelled 'In bits of love, my heart'.

I felt that today he was using Butch (and Pierre) to protect himself from too close a contact with me, but did not interpret this.

104th Session (Saturday 2.4.55)

S. – I had another dream last night. I was with Ginette in the metro, the underneath part, and she was with her special girl friend, who once saved her life. I was very jealous because I was not with Butch. At that moment I found myself here with you and I was doing a drawing of a bottom doing BMs. What does that mean?

J. M. – Perhaps there is an idea that you would like to do BMs here with me? And it may be that you think Ginette and her girl friend do it together.

S. – Yes I often wonder what they do. Is that what they do?

J. M. – It might also have something to do with things you'd like to do with Butch.

S. – Ummm, um! Oh, that Ginette, she's so fat and juicy. I would like to be right inside that girl.

J. M. – You would like to get right inside her bottom?

S. – Well, uh, perhaps. I used to worry such a lot about bottoms, especially very round bottoms, but now I don't think about it any more. By the way, have you noticed that I don't play with the animals any more? I wonder why that is?

J. M. – Perhaps it has something to do with BMs and bottoms too.

S. – You know, Dougie, I think I'm getting a lot better. Before, I couldn't talk about such things if I didn't have animals and stories, and now I don't *have* to any more. I can just talk to you like we're doing now. It's so much easier. And you know, I never get bored now. Everything goes so quickly. Do you think my troubles are getting better? Oh and there's something else that troubles me. When will I get over worrying what my parents do? I mean, when I'm not there.

J. M. – What sort of things do they do?

176

S. – Oh, at night. I don't know. When they're still in the lounge and I'm in bed.

J. M. – Perhaps you feel that your parents are doing exciting things together and that makes you feel left out.

S. – Oh, but my parents don't do *that*. You might do things with *your* husband, but they just talk. (In an anxious tone.) Do you think that's all they do, Dougie?

J. M. – What's really important is what you think they do.

S. – I have a second worry too and that's the penis and breast trouble.

J. M. – What is that exactly?

S. – Well, about me wanting to have breasts, and I'm always so afraid about my penis too.

J. M. – It sounds as though you would like to be both sexes and not just one. Can you tell me a bit more about it?

S. – Well, I'll get a lot of hair around it, but I don't know when. Will it come out slowly? Will it prickle me?

Sammy then asks what I am going to think of him when he is thirty years old, and he wants details about the things we shall do on the last day of his analysis. I attach these fantasies to the fact that this is the last day before a three-weeks Easter break and that it also concerns his thoughts about himself as the man he will become. He then expresses considerable anxiety about the holiday break, and is able to accept that not only does he fear the separation but in addition his concern about his parents' sexual activity is partly stimulated by the idea that I shall be alone with my husband and may forget about him during the holidays.

105th Session (Thursday 21.4.55)

Sammy gives a detailed and for once entirely coherent account of his holiday. The most exciting event was that he met a very nice lady who was in charge of the desk at the hotel and with whom he fell in love. In addition, he found a boy of his own age and managed to play with him. He then adds that he had some interesting conversations with his mother about Sigmund Freud.

Mrs Y had telephoned me to say that the Special School seemed eager to accept Sammy and that the Director would be in Paris in two weeks.

106th Session (Friday 22.4.55)

Sammy begins talking about the Director of the American School, complaining that he doesn't want to see him and doesn't want to leave Paris. While recounting these things, he breaks off suddenly.

> S. – Dougie, I have an important thought, but I wonder what would happen to me if I told you.

He searches around for different ways of approaching this thought.

> S. – Oh, it's so hard to explain. It's when I look out of the window. I fell something terrible is going to happen. Then I look up and see that all the buildings are smiling, and on days when I feel happy and gay, the buildings all look very serious. But they sometimes look serious when I'm sad, too. Oh, I don't know, everything looks so sad most of the time to me. All the things in the street, everything looks at me sadly.
>
> J. M. – Perhaps these are bits of your own feeling that you've put on to the buildings and things outside you.
>
> S. – This worries me. Do other people have these ideas too? It's bad, isn't it?
>
> J. M. – You seem to think that to have feelings is bad.
>
> S. – Yes, I do! Is it alright to feel things? Oh, and there's something else I want to ask you. Does this happen to other people? Let's say I'm looking at the drawing of a boy I don't like at school. His drawing always looks angry back at me. But my own drawing always look happy at me. And when I'm walking in the street, people's coats say, 'Ha, ha, you can't have me. I belong here on this person, but not on you!' This doesn't happen to me with people I love. My mother's clothes always look so happy, and sometimes a man's sleeve can look happy, but Dougie, I *know* these things aren't living.
>
> J. M. – Well, I think it's something like this. You're afraid of all these live and strong feelings when they're inside you, and so you put them outside instead.
>
> S. – Ah—ha! Well, there's another thing too. (Sammy talks quickly and anxiously as though he were afraid there would not be enough time.) I don't know why it interests me because it's not really a *bad* thing. It's the way the roof of the train curves. I just keep staring and staring at it. And then I'm always kissing the girls at school, too. Is that bad?

J. M. – What do you think?

S. – No, it isn't! But I do bad things to them. I slap them because I want to see them cry. Is that a happy way of loving do you think? Why do I do it? Will I ever get over it? Do adults do it? . . . I'm so afraid I'm going to grow up to be a coward. I'm afraid of what people will do to me.

J. M. – Perhaps it's a bit like the angry drawing. You put the inside feeling outside, so that what you are really afraid of is what you might want to do to others.

S. – Yes, I know that's true! But is that being a coward all the same? Do any other people feel these things? Oh yes, and there's another thing. I sometimes imagine that my house is going up and down, and it's just as though I'm watching it in a mirror. Is it bad? Is there anything wrong with it?

It is clear from the way in which Sammy talks about this fantasy that it is quite different in quality from that of the buildings which are crying or smiling. I say to him that there are many ways of imagining things; that many people do it, and we call it 'day-dreaming' because we realise that these things are not true. Sammy is most interested and happy to hear this.

In this session, particularly at the beginning, Sammy's 'personalisation' of the external world takes on a psychotic quality. To give a face and a language to the outside world is a megalomanic defence which denies and annuls the little boy's impotence in the face of my twice-repeated rejection (the Easter holidays and his departure for America). It is only a step from the fantasies Sammy is expressing to certain delusional ideas in adults.

Later, when the interpretation is made that Sammy wants to avoid some of his feelings, the internal depersonalisation and the external cathexis give the impression of a new defence along obsessional lines. Sammy alludes, as in the 95th Session, to the curved roof of the train. Here he does not bestow life on the train, instead he endows it with a deep symbolic signifi-cance. That is, it seems to him less dangerous to have imaginary relationships without obvious significance; it is simpler to think of the back of a train than of a woman's behind. This process of displacement and denial will not allay his anxiety completely, and the energy of the drive attached to the new symbolic object will cathect the obsessive fantasies with the same dangers he sought to avoid. It is none the less true that in a psychotic structure, this neuroticising of the ego allows a measure of control over anxiety, and may avoid, to some extent, the use of delusional projection as a defence.

107th Session (Saturday 23.4.55)

Sammy talks a lot about the American School, then jumps towards my chair, throws his arms around my neck, kissing me and pummelling me. On my insisting that he verbalise rather than act out his feelings, he sits down.

S. – Do you mind if you have a baby? You might have one after what I just did to you!

J. M. – What was it you did exactly?

S. – When I kissed you I pushed my stomach into your what's-it.

J. M. – Is that what would make the baby?

S. – Oh, you don't have to take your clothes off, you know (in a very uncertain tone of voice), do you? What is it they do really? You can keep your clothes on, I know you can, my mother told me so—sometimes, that is. But it's in bed that you do it. What is it that I have to do to you to make a baby?

J. M. – Tell me what you think happens.

S. – I know, I'll *draw* it for you.

Sammy then draws a picture of a man with a rather large, erect penis, and of a woman with an extremely small dent opposite this penis. He then asks dozens of questions: How does the penis get in? Does it get out all right? Why is it sometimes big and why is it sometimes small?

J. M. – I expect you're talking about your own penis.

S. – Oh yes. It used to happen to me when I was little. I used to put my hands around it. I didn't like it like that when it got big. Tell me, does the baby come out of the father's penis? Oh, there are so many interesting questions? Can a man do peepee inside a woman? And where exactly is this hole of hers? What happens to the man's seeds if he doesn't put them inside her? How does the baby get out? How does the milk get to the baby?

As far as possible, I try to get Sammy to elaborate on his fantasies, and reassure him on the points where it is obvious that he already knows the answers.

S. – May I ask some more questions? How does food get through our bodies, and how does it get turned into BMs and peepee?

J. M. – Well, we don't have any more time today to talk about it, but you can tell me next time what you think about it.

Following his 'sexual exchange' with me, Sammy is effectively reassured that the playing-out of his fantasy does not produce any kind of catastrophe, and it is possibly this factor which permitted him to ask a number of objective questions about sexual relationships.

108th Session (Monday 25.4.55)

Sammy talks again about the house going up and down and the buildings which cry when he is happy and laugh when he is sad. He then recounts an incident which happened this morning. Mme R, one of the assistants at the school, suddenly smacked him without warning, because he had been annoying the girls. Sammy was thoroughly indignant at this injustice and says he bit her hand until it bled. He then goes on to describe what he will do to her if she ever tries this again. He imagines a series of savage attacks and ends up with '. . . and I'll smash her, just until her head rolls between her legs'. At this point he jumps suddenly to his feet, throws his arms around me from the back of my chair and begins kissing me and violently thrusts his hands into my blouse, then seizes my earrings. I point out that he has made his sudden attack upon me at the moment of telling about the school teacher, thus stimulating his fears of attack from women.

J. M. – And when you grab at my blouse and take my earrings, it's as though you want to get something back from me for yourself. You grabbed at my breasts as though you're still afraid that I want to take away your penis.

S. – Have you seen Dr Lebovici recently? I wonder how *he's* getting on.

J. M. – You think I've taken his penis too?

S. – Yeah, I do!

181

Sammy calms down and pulls his chair over beside mine, but he continues to smack me, blow kisses at me and pull at my clothing.

S. – Dougie, you're a beautiful, kind mother. What do other patients do here with you? What would people say if they saw what I'm doing?

J. M. – You're wondering if this is the way grown-up people behave together. If this is the way your father is with your mother?

S. – If your husband came in now, would he think you didn't love him any more? (Sammy is blowing on me at this moment.)

J. M. – Perhaps you would like to take me away from my husband? When you said just now that I was a beautiful, kind mother, maybe you were thinking you would like to do these things with your mother and take her away from Daddy?

At this moment Sammy goes and sits quietly in his chair. He then recounts an incident which occurred yesterday in which his father became extremely angry with the waiter in a café because the service was bad. (My interpretation of the desires directed to his mother has the effect of calling to mind the angry father.)

109th Session (Tuesday 26.4.55)

Sammy is very angry throughout the session and spends his time hitting me, and intermittently demands to be served with drinks, milk, fruit juice, water. I tell him that he is perhaps identifying himself with the angry father of whom he talked during the last session. At the same time, when he demands drinks, he is no doubt making an oral demand for the restitution of his phallic power, which he feels is concealed in me.

110th Session (Thursday 28.4.55)

Most of the session is devoted to the 'day-dreams', of which I noted only one or two examples.

S. – Today it happened again. I was having lunch at school and I suddenly saw the table whizzing past. It's another day-dream, isn't it?

J. M. – Was there anything that happened at the table to upset you?

S. – Oh yes, there was. There was a visitor. A deaf lady. I couldn't stop looking at her. Gee, I was scared of her!

I explain Sammy's projective fantasy to him as something which might happen when he is anxious, and which represents his desire to pitch anxious thoughts outside of himself. (With Sammy's urgent need to project everything, and feel it is being *taken in*, a deaf person would be as frightening to him as a deaf analyst.) He talks again of the houses and buildings looking sad, and says he has talked this matter over with his father.

S. – Please don't think I imagine he knows more than you. I think you know more. Well, I don't know, but it's a big difficulty for me.

J. M. – I expect you would like me to be a sort of father for you some-times, but at other times you need to feel that Daddy is stronger than me.

S. – Well, about the buildings, maybe it's because I don't *like* to feel happy. What do you think? Oh, and there's another trouble too; my father talked to me about it. Have you noticed that I talk in a funny way very often?

(Sammy does frequently talk in a very bizarre fashion, using automatic phrases with little apparent meaning, strings of inap-propriate clichés interspersed with shrieks and barking noises.)

J. M. – Yes, sometimes you use a sort of 'special talking'. Can you tell me more about it yourself.

S. – I do it nearly all the time with my father. It makes him very mad at me. And I do it to my sister too. My mother keeps telling me to stop it, but I can't. I only do it to people I know well. Oh, Dougie, I do want to stop it! What can I do? And there's another thing. I want to stop hitting the girls and wanting to see them cry. You must get this trouble away from me. About the day-dreams, I don't mind, because it's only me that's bothered, but these other things that hurt people, how can I stop that? I don't really like hurting other people. Can you help me, Dougie? You see, I'm talking quite natur-ally now, aren't I?

In the preceding session, the oedipal interpretation pro-voked a lively resistance which is manifested in the deperson-alised material of this session. The regression caused by oedipal guilt leads to the psychotic world of which Sammy becomes more and more consciously aware when he says that he does not like to feel happy and that he sometimes talks in a crazy way, that is, an autistic type of isolation. Rather than fight with girls, which means play out with them condemned sexual activities, he prefers to live in his dream world where he is alone and can harm no one.

Theories about psychosis generally stress the importance of pre-genital fantasies, but frequently there is confusion between pre-genital and pre-oedipal, as this session illustrates. From the beginning, oedipal guilt feelings were evident. The oscillations between a genitalised oedipal situation, and a situation charged with pre-genital fantasies, are represented in Sammy by a subtle interplay of fantasies which are built up one on top of the other, or which are set up as defences against each other.

Sammy's search for paternal protection against oedipal guilt feelings is again in evidence.

111th Session (Friday 22.4.55)

Sammy is again in a very aggressive mood, but makes obvious attempts to control it. After trying to hit me, he suddenly sits down.

S. – I haven't told you yet that when I'm in the toilet it's funny too. Sometimes I look at the top of the toilet and it seems either sad or happy, and then I know what the day will be like and whether I'll be happy or sad.

Sammy makes a rapid sketch of the toilet looking happy and the toilet looking sad.

S. – And sometimes it smells a bit sick, and again after someone has been there, there's a big worry for me. Oh, but you won't help me. I wish I could have been analysed by Sigmund Freud or Dr Mahler, or Anna Freud. I'm sure they're better than you.

Sammy jumps towards me and hits out at me, at the same time fondling and blowing down my neck.

S. – Oh, I think I smell something down there. Did you make a fart-fart?

J. M. – Bad things coming out of me?

Sammy tries to scratch and bite and I put him firmly back into his seat and tell him to talk about it instead.

S. – Well, I want to see what you've got.

J. M. – You want to know what's inside me?

S. – Yes, I'm going to see!

J. M. – You can make a drawing of it, and that way we'll understand it together.

Sammy then makes a 'portrait' of me commenting all the while. (Fig. 7.)

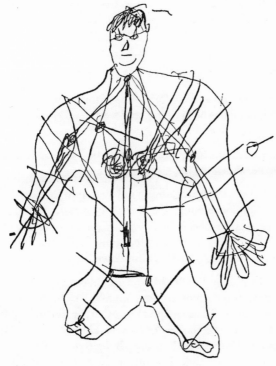

Fig. 7

S. – Your bones are made of metal, and no one can see. And the skin slides, it's not like mine. Now here your bones are attached with elastic, and there are your breasts, shining like two lights. You have no heart, you aren't special enough for that! You've just a little brick.

185

Sammy has great difficulty with the drawing of my backbone. While struggling with this problem of perspective, he leans over from time to time and hits me on the arms. At one point he also demands that I draw his 'insides' but does not insist. I ask him what we would find in his insides. He comes over to my chair and alternatively hits, kisses and bites me, and mumbles 'mummy, mummma, mummmy, mummmma'.

J. M. – Is that what you want to do with your mother?

He hits me again, but does not sit down. All his talk is incoherent, and reminds me of his first weeks of analysis. Clearly I am the 'heartless' analyst who will neither satisfy his love demands nor protect him.

112th Session (Saturday 30.4.55)

Sammy again asks Hélène for a glass of milk. He talks about some clay modelling he has been doing, and says that he has just finished a model of Jesus's grave.

> S. – His real grave, and, and, oh my ladies! Oh my lee. Oh he . . .
> He, he, eh, eh . . .

For the first time I draw Sammy's attention to the fact that he has lapsed into 'special talking'. He looks very crossly at me, and I tell him that he is angry because I am touching one of his protective devices, and remind him that yesterday he was afraid of bad things coming out of me. He suddenly calms down.

> S. – Oh, I think that's why I had a dream last night. I dreamt that there was something coming out of my right side. It was some stuff, like two hands gripped together, or something. I wanted to touch it and to feel the bones. Then a voice said: 'Don't touch the bones!' Is there any thought in this dream?
> J. M. – Perhaps you think I want to stop you touching things? Especially to stop you touching what comes out of yourself. Your penis or your behind.

Sammy leans over and smacks me, but at the same moment recalls another dream from last night in which he is in a forest with a small, black dog. He hears his father at the back of the house, and his father asks why he is making a noise. He gives a number of curious associations to this dream, and then tells me that he made it up. He then remembers a dream where someone was crying behind some bushes. He woke up and found it was his baby sister. He also recalls another dream in which an unknown person was being very cruel to Ginette.

S.–I must tell you that yesterday I had a trouble when I walked past a building that some men are working on. They work so slowly. It's quite different where I come from, but the trouble was I had a thought as I went by. (Sammy looks very embarrassed at this moment.) I said the words, 'Oh, the poor metro won't be able to get by.' It's a bit silly, isn't it, Dougie? I know the metro isn't alive, but I do get worried when I think that they'll never get that building finished.

J. M.–Perhaps the worry about getting things finished has got something to do with worrying about not finishing your analysis with me, since we know that you may have to go back to America.

S.–That's a horrible worry. I won't think about it! I wonder why I think the metro is alive.

J. M.–Well, you talked about it before as though you felt it were part of you, when you told me you mustn't touch it. You remember you thought it was wrong even to play the metro game, like touching the bones in your dream? It's like another way of worrying about your penis as you often do.

S.–Oh yes. It isn't that silly, to worry about the metro, is it?

Sammy jumps up and kisses me, and then goes back to his chair. He then tells a story about a man in his house who does everything for him and 'fixes him up'. He starts to ask many questions about other patients, but becomes increasingly restless and again comes over to hit me and kiss me. I put him firmly back in his chair and tell him he must talk about it instead.

S.–Oh, I like a psychoanalyst who is severe with me!

J. M.–Yes, I think you often do these things so that I will prevent you.

S.–But I wish you'd be really *cruel* to me like the Pharaoh whipping the Hebrews.

He comes over to my chair whispering, 'I love you, I love you' and hitting me at the same time. At one moment he grabs a pencil and makes as though to stab me with it. I draw back.

S. – Oh you don't love me else you wouldn't be afraid of me. (He climbs on to the back of my chair and puts his head on my shoulder.) Let's just continue our psychoanalysis like this. Now we're cooking with gas. I have another trouble to tell you.

I tell him to go back to his chair and talk about his trouble but he continues pulling at my clothing and my hair and finally has the idea of piling cushions on my head. When I tell him that this isn't getting us anywhere he says, 'How come you're so severe today?' His provocative heaping of cushions upon me finally wins out and he clearly wants me to play a forbidding paternal role. I am fed up and say very crossly, 'Sammy I'm sick of this. Now you just sit down!' He immediately settles back into his chair and makes a drawing.

S. – This is an island. All is silent around like in Israel, and the sea is quiet. Suddenly this 'thing' happens. (He draws brisk lines shooting out of his island.) The people get so surprised they go crazy. What has happened? Is it a day-dream?

J. M. – When does all this happen?

S. – It's 4 o'clock in the daytime. (He adds in a drawing of a clock marking 4 and is astounded when I remind him that this is the time of his sessions.)

J. M. – Also you have just provoked me into getting angry. Maybe you would like something dramatic to happen between us. You know those lines shooting out of your island are exactly the same as the ones you did the other day in the fire drawing. You told me they were fire lines and that they stood for love. Perhaps this is a day-dream about some kind of violent loving you would like to share with me?

S. – Oh Dougie it's a bit true. I do like the idea of you're being cruel and it's very exciting.

J. M. – A bit like the spanks you used to get from your mother?

S. – Yes, and that reminds me of another day-dream. I often think about the metros rushing into one another and crashing and I get so excited. You know, Dougie, I think I'm getting some of these troubles out of my head. Do you think I'm doing alright?

He goes off euphorically and I note after the session that Sammy clearly wants to make me into the complete 'positive' oedipal couple. He wants to make a violent pre-genital love to me as the mother and at the same time wants me to play the forbidding oedipal father who will prevent any realisation of these incestuous wishes. In this respect he is also seeking a strong masculine figure with whom to identify, and he tries to locate this person inside me. At that moment Sammy rushes back into the consulting-room and whispers, 'I caught a glimpse. Hélène has just shown in a woman patient of yours. Those two are no good. They have no . . .' and he points to his penis.

The manifest content of Sammy's dream recalls the drawing of the previous session. A very primitive oedipal situation might be suggested here, the penis being compared to the analyst's inside and erection thought to be the result of the wish to possess the good food in there. The disembodied voice forbids this, but it is not until Sammy recounts the invented dream that the father is introduced—apparently to forbid masturbation. This latter situation suggests an oedipal structure with a recently developed identification with the aggressor. In the last part of the session where Sammy wants a cruel and severe analyst he succeeds in finding the father in the mother he desires. On this basis he develops a masochistic fantasy in which the mother is imagined as behaving sadistically, and this is secondarily eroticised.

113th Session (Monday 2.5.55)

S.-I have a trouble to tell you. Today I was playing at trains again. Is it very bad? Sometimes I do it all afternoon, and I make the noise that they make going into the tunnel.

I sum up all that has been said recently about trains, and interpret Sammy's anxiety about his game as one relative to primal scene fantasies and the noises associated.

S.-All that, yeah. Sometimes my parents stop it. I don't think that worries me. But I've never seen them do it. Would they ever let me watch? Would you let your sons watch, even if I didn't make any noise?

I make unsuccessful attempts to encourage Sammy to tell me what he would expect to see.

S. – Well, I suppose I'll just have to wait until I have a wife of my own. I want lots of sons and daughters. I might have a hundred of them, and I'm going to bring all my sons over here to show you. When my troubles are finished. Is it alright to have a hundred sons?

J. M. – You want to make lots more than your daddy? (Sammy grins with pleasure, but now modifies his fantasy.)

S. – If you saw my wife with a black dress on, what would you think about her? Can white people marry black people?

J. M. – Thinking of Butch?

S. – Yes. You know, Dougie, he hasn't even written to me and I wrote such a nice letter, and I look every day for his letter.

J. M. – Have you noticed that often when you talk about having a wife or being with women you start right away to think about Butch? Perhaps thinking about Butch makes you less worried than thinking about girls and women, and yourself being a father one day.

S. – Ya, ya, I know all about that. Now that's enough of that; I want to tell you about Butch.

Sammy finds many reasons which might explain the lack of news from Butch. He talks in a very normal, rational way until the end of the session.

The cathexis of inanimate objects and toys is such that symbolic function is lost; the train-game is no longer symbolic but becomes real. In the same way, at the beginning of the analysis, language itself was cathected thus preventing words from exercising their function of communication. The cognitive processes are invaded by an anxiety which the ego is unable to cope with. Even though Sammy has made great progress in these areas, and has been able to free important sectors of ego activity, it is none the less true that this cathexis of the external world is a serious obstacle.

114th Session (Tuesday 3.5.55)

Sammy asks Hélène for a glass of water. He then recounts a day-dream. A boy in the street rushes up and kills Sammy's father. In great anger, Sammy pushes the boy over, and knocks him into a sewer. Sammy begins balancing the glass of water back and forth, obviously with the intention of throwing it should I begin to talk. He breaks into a spate of 'special talking'—a stream of gibberish, automatic phrases, squeals and grunts. His excitement mounts rapidly, and my interpretations go unheard. I lean over to take the glass of water from him and he throws it all over the wall. My countertransference gets the better of me, and I speak crossly to him. Sammy immediately looks terrified. He creeps over to my chair and then sits on my lap. I explain to him just what has been happening in the last few minutes, his fear of the fantasy about the boy who killed his father and his reasons for wanting to throw the water over me, as if to kill my husband.

> S.–And did you notice the 'special talking'? Why do I do that, Dougie? I do it a lot here, don't I? But it's much worse when I'm with my father.
>
> J. M.–Yes, there must be some special reason for that. You say it makes your father very angry when you do it. We know you do it when you are very worried about your thoughts. Do you think you may also do it to punish your father a little bit?
>
> S.–Oh, I never thought of that! Maybe I'll get over this one day. And why did I throw the water? I wish I hadn't! And you know, I wouldn't do it now.
>
> J. M.–Well, why do you think you did it?
>
> S.–I just got too excited to stop.
>
> J. M.–Yes, and the 'special talking' is also when you are afraid of all your excitement, and all of the feelings and noises that come out of you—or your parents. Like the excitement today over your day-dream.
>
> S.–Please tell me more about my excitements. I must get them all away.

I show Sammy that the fantasy of the boy who kills his father is very frightening because of his own fear of his aggressive thoughts towards his father, coupled with fears of revenge, of being disposed of anally, like the boy who was pushed into the sewer. Then the thoughts about the trains, and the frightening connection between killing and sexual fantasy. Sammy is so intensely interested in this explanation that we go on to all the noises he produces in his special talking. I show him that many of them are fart-fart noises, which he uses in order to expel the frightening fantasies. Sammy is nevertheless still hurt by my having said that throwing water was no great progress and that he could have talked about it instead. I tell him that I was cross because of my own excitements and feelings, but that even so, he had managed to get his fantasy out, and after all it was a very frightening one. Sammy then reviews all the 'progress' which he has accomplished up to now: he is much less afraid to go for walks on his own, gets on better with other children, is working well at school. (So in general he is more interested in the outside world than in his fascinating, but terrifying inner world.)

115th Session (Thursday 5.5.55)

S. – I dreamt last night I was sitting here with you, and I suddenly found that I was all naked. I wasn't a bit ashamed—I just felt a little bit cold. Something interesting happened yesterday. My sister had an X-ray. She was all naked from the waist down. I like seeing her naked.

J. M. – In your dream, you were all naked too. Perhaps you would also like to be looked at by the doctors and by me?

S. – Yes! Is it bad?

J. M. – Perhaps you are pleased that you have a penis and your sister doesn't. Maybe you are saying that it's quite safe to have a penis and yet be here with me. (I think Sammy also feels 'naked' because we have been 'uncovering' so many of his defences, the special talking, etc.)

S. – That reminds me of something that I want to explain. It's very hard, but you'll understand. I'm sure no one else would. It's when I'm waiting for the metro. I get very bothered if the metro doesn't come right out of the tunnel. I like it best when it comes right out and goes beyond the 'tête de train' notice.

J. M. – What do you think worries you about that?

S. – Oh, it has to do with BMs. I know, it's constipation! I like everything in certain positions, and when they don't get into the right positions, it's a big trouble. I like to stare at the windows in churches because they're so regular, and when you lie down in a boat and I look at the front part dead-on, the lines run together.

Sammy went on to give innumerable examples of his preoccupations with lines, perspective, numbers and letters. I noted only a few of these afterwards. For example, the importance of certain numbers. '3' is a good number for Sammy. He describes it as 'solid, safe and reliable'. '1' is terrible; '2' and '0' have something disturbing about them. He hopes one day he will like the number '4'. The letters of the alphabet are also highly invested. 'E' is an especially good letter, because it is strong and has the '3' in it. 'A' is like two legs. There 'is something a bit wrong with it, but on the whole it is alright'. 'O' is not alright at all. 'R' is alright because it combines the two things, 'E' and 'O'. I ask Sammy whether he thinks that all these feelings about the letters and numbers are connected with his ideas about people's bodies and that the number '3' in particular perhaps reminds him of masculine genitals and makes him feel that it is protective.

Sammy is in a state of elation throughout the session and hardly stops talking for one moment, as if he has to talk fast in order to get all these ideas out into the open. He asks me to write down everything we have talked about, to be careful to forget nothing and to make a note that he has much more to say about 'cars and boats coming to a point' (i.e. perspective). He asks politely if he may have a sheet of paper to illustrate his fascination with perspective, and he actually uses it for this purpose, which is in marked contrast to his previous behaviour where he always had to have at least twenty sheets and rarely managed to express, in a clear way, ideas of this sort.

The following day, due to some muddle-up at home, which had nothing to do with Sammy, he was unable to come to his session. He telephoned to explain what had happened, and was most disturbed and unhappy about it all.

The atmosphere of the session indicates the presence of a number of defence mechanisms which express the newly evolving ego-organisation already discussed. The interpretation of castration anxiety releases an immediate association to an obsessive idea about the metro. The latter is seen as a phallic appendage, but this symbolic image is now charged with anxiety and takes on an obsessive character. The engine must pass a certain point. It goes without saying that this anxiety is infinitely better controlled that that aroused by projective fusion with the external world, in the fight against dissociation. The anal fixations serve to keep the symbolic object at a distance, and Sammy is then able to talk of the metro as an anal penis. In a way which is quasi-experimental, and somewhat surprising, he then goes on to talk of his concern for order and symmetry, and the symbolic value which he attaches to letters and numbers. Inanimate letters take on a representative value and are invested with living and *conscious* significance. It is not surprising that Sammy has until recently found it impossible to learn to read or write!

116th Session (Saturday 7.5.55)

Sammy asks immediately for the drawing he has made of churches in perspective and for the notes of last Thursday's session. He then goes on to tell me that he touched the train today on the curved bit at the back end. He describes the incident in terms of great excitement and also great shame.

> S. – I wouldn't want anyone to see me doing that. They'd think I was nuts!

Sammy makes a connection between the excitement he feels over the back curve of the trains and the perspective of two cars passing one another. He gives many instances of this kind of excitement.

> S. – Now, I must tell you about two dreams I had. I was with my father and there was a whole string of churches behind us. My father and I go through an archway, and then I am all alone. Away ahead of me I saw a deer coming towards me. When it got closer it turned into a yak, and when it got right up close, I saw it was a rhino coming at me. It was horrible and I was frightened when I woke up.

Sammy becomes very anxious when I ask him what he thinks about rhinos. He leans over and hits me, but at the same time, brings up a number of associations connected with the film 'Ivory Hunters' which he had talked about several months ago.

> S. – But these ideas are all finished with! I don't think like that any more, and now that'll do. Don't let's talk about it or I'll hit you!
>
> J. M. – If this dream makes you feel so angry there must be something frightening in it, so let's talk about it anyway.

194

I put together various ideas from earlier sessions and interpret his dream as representative of conflict with his father, in connection with his desire to be close to me and at the same time his intense fear in the face of this desire; and that this fear is connected with the fantasies of being destroyed by his father's penis. He would like to have his father's strength, but this carries lots of dangers with it.

S. – Well, maybe it has something to do with the second dream too. I was being chased through the house by a kind of lion or tiger. I kept shutting the doors, but it got through all the time.

J. M. – Does that dream make you think of anything in particular?

S. – Yes, my mother! I was afraid she'd be so angry with me because I missed my session. When she came home I hid behind the door.

(Sammy here talks as though his missing the session was his own fault. This was purely imaginary; his mother had herself explained by telephone the extraneous circumstances.)

J. M. – Well, it seems as though in your dream you're saying that you have to be afraid of your mother because she might eat you up if you don't do what she expects and maybe you were afraid I'd be angry too because you didn't come. But I think it has something to do with the ideas in the first dream too, of wanting to get close to your father and thinking that your mother will be angry with you for that. You have to keep shutting the doors as though you have to protect your penis and your behind.

S. – I wish I knew why I have to keep touching things. Is it bad? I keep thinking it's wrong.

I link this feeling to the idea of touching trains, and interpret his feeling that it is forbidden to touch his body, that he is actually aware of feeling, above all, that he must not touch his bottom, but that he probably means his penis.

S. – How do you know that I touch my penis? Oh, I want to touch the trains so badly I don't know what to do. It seems to come out towards me, and I seem to have to touch it.

J. M. – Like the rhinoceros?

S. – (As though he has recovered a certain gleam of memory.) Oh yes, that was part of it! Yes, when I was very little I couldn't stop drawing rhinos. And then there were horses too. I remember once when I was at holiday camp two years ago and I saw the horses touch bottoms, two of them together. I wanted to touch the bottom of the horse and to feel it all alive and warm and I wanted to put my head against it. Then one horse farted on the other. I was so jealous, I wanted to be the other horse.

I trace for Sammy the link between present compulsive ideas about touching trains etc. back to his memory of the horse. Sammy is very struck by this.

> S. – But that's much better, isn't it? I thought it was bad to go on liking horses. It's better to feel something about a horse than about a train, isn't it?
>
> J. M. – Of course. It's much more alive.
>
> S. – Oh, how wonderful. Everything is wonderful today!

He goes off delightedly. Sammy was to tell me later what an important place rhinos had in his fantasy life when he was seven or eight years old. For a whole year, he did nothing but draw rhinos and make up stories about them. (In the phase of his analysis where he played the animal games he avoided touching the rhinos.)

> 'My father and I go through an archway together' suggests a symbolic penetration of the mother together — a supportive identification. But once through, Sammy is all alone, and it is then that he meets the frightening rhino-penis charging towards him. The second dream surges into Sammy's mind when I talk of his wish to take in his father's strength. Here he is shutting doors against an angry devouring animal which he himself associates with his mother. In part constructed from his own projections or oral wishes, this image is also undoubtedly connected with his homosexual wish for the father's penis, probably imagined as an anal introjection. He shuts the doors as a defence against this wish. It is also highly possible that much of Sammy's masturbation has been anal rather than phallic.
>
> We can see that Sammy's ego has been considerably enriched since he is now able to express a fantasy of the primal scene through a screen memory — the horses touching behinds

and farting. The integration of this past experience at this moment in the analysis gives Sammy a happy optimistic feeling about sexual desires and loving, as realms which might be possible for him after all.

117th Session (Monday 9.5.55)

Sammy demands milk from Hélène as soon as he comes into the waiting-room. Having drunk the milk, he hits me, and thrusts his hands down the neck of my frock. I put together his need to have things from inside me in the form of drinking milk, and his feeling that I am hiding my husband's penis there. Sammy grabs my earrings and makes as if to throw them away.

J. M. – Dangerous bits of me that you want to throw far away?

Sammy comes and drops them into my hands, and demands that I praise him for being so co-operative. At the same moment, he kisses me and blows down my neck.

S. – My father says male analysts are the best!

(He then goes on to talk of the special school in America and expresses great concern at having to discuss all his problems with another analyst. He spends much of the session on this theme and his distress about having to leave Paris in a few months. He says it would be impossible for him to talk about the fart-fart to anybody else. He comes over and embraces me and immediately says that male analysts will be much better for him. I point out his need for paternal protection in relation to a woman. This immediately brings up once more his preoccupation with touching and his intense desire to touch trains, horses, etc.

J. M. – And rhinos?
S. – Yes, rhinos most of all. It's the skin and the horn, but I was always so afraid he would push it into me. Oh, oh, I cannot go to another analyst!! It would be too hard to tell. Would another analyst understand about the rhino? Anyway, it's not such a great trouble now. But I have another trouble. You said that I was making along well when I could say the troubles out. Is it bad that I don't seem to have so many any more? I never talk about my insides and my appendix ache. I

don't seem to think about that any more and I don't get the heart pains either. But can we talk about it tomorrow?

118th Session (Tuesday 10.5.55)

Sammy is again very preoccupied with trains and returns incessantly to the question, but why do I *touch* it? I recapitulate the chain of displacements, from backs of trains to backs of horses, to rhinos and their horns, to penis, to father. Sammy refuses this interpretation, probably because he feels that an important defence is threatened. In any case, my interpretation brings no modification of his compulsive questioning.

He goes on to explain the importance of standing in the metro and looking *down* on to the next compartment. He says this excites him enormously, but it worries him because he doesn't understand it. He compares it to a feeling of comfort and protection as when he is sitting in a big chair and can look down on people in smaller chairs.

J. M. – Perhaps it's a way of feeling safer?

S. – Yes, I don't like things that are higher than me.

J. M. – What sort of things?

S. – Breasts. They're higher than my penis!

Sammy then plays out a game in which he constantly bumps into my chair and sometimes into me. Apart from the breast-penis situation, my chair also is a little higher than his. After a bit he suddenly returns to his chair, looking sheepish, and saying he feels upset. I ask him about this, and he tells me that he has just realised he is being very babyish.

S. – I want to tell you about two troubles that are hard to explain. It's really just a feeling I have. It's not a thought, more like an idea in my head. It could be a dream, but it isn't because I'm awake. Everything suddenly sometimes seems sort of far off. But it isn't, it's still there. People around me are all tiny. Of course they're just as usual, I suppose, but they seem different. It's a terrible trouble. Do you know about this trouble?

J. M. – When does this kind of trouble seem to come about?

S. – It happened the other day when my father was explaining about chain-letters to me. He went on talking and I couldn't understand anything, and it was very frightening. And the other trouble is that I'm often seeing things but not looking.

198

I suggest to Sammy that we name these sensations of depersonal-isation, 'the dream-feeling', and tell him we will talk about it at the next session. I make a note to tell him that these troubled-feelings started up today after the talk about breasts and penis as though he thought it were better to become Dougie-with-biting-breasts than Sammy-whose-penis-is threatened. His feelings of fright about being himself have something to do with bringing on the 'dream-feeling', and losing a solid feeling of his own identity.

119th Session (Thursday 12.5.55)

After discussing yesterday's session Sammy talks of his anxiety about leaving Paris and having a new analyst.

> S. – I got the 'dream-feeling' again yesterday when I had to go and see the doctor. Does anybody else have this trouble? Does it go on very long? I don't think it's possible to stand it for long. It feels awful. Do you know what it's like, Dougie? Please tell me more about the other patients.

Sammy discusses what he thinks other patients do here. Up to the end of the session he talks in a normal voice and expresses his ideas logically, like any boy of his age. Today he is to go home alone, since his mother is not able to come and collect him as she usually does. Going out, he says, 'I want to kiss you goodbye', and follows this by kissing me very gently on the neck. He immediately breaks into a stream of squeals and grunts.

> S. – Oh look, I'm 'special talking' again. I didn't make any of those fart-fart noises until now, but I'm still doing quite a lot of it at home. I wonder why I did it just now?

I suggest to Sammy that it is linked with his desire to kiss me good-bye and the fact that his mother is not here. (That is, the 'special talking' is produced in place of a fantasy, and helps to keep the fantasy unconscious.)

120th Session (Friday 13.5.55)

> S. – Dougie, please smell my hands. I've been touching the trains again; can you smell it?
> J. M. – We were talking the other day about touching trains and touching bottoms being something alike. Maybe you think your hands have a bottom smell.

S. – But I don't touch bottoms any more. Oh yes, I do, in the bath. I love to soap my bottom a lot and I put lots around my penis too, and my armpits and neck.

(Sammy's mother has complained about Sammy's excessive bathing and soaping. It is no doubt a defence against masturbation.)

S. – (Pulling a handkerchief out of his pocket.) This handkerchief belongs to my teacher's husband, and I blow my nose in it all the time. It's much better than the paper handkerchiefs that you give to me to blow my nose on.

J. M. – I expect you feel safer with Monsieur Dupont's handkerchief.

S. – Yes. It's like a bit of him. I feel like we were touching noses.

J. M. – Like touching bottoms?

S. – The real trouble is that I've had no letter from Butch!

Although I don't at this point interpret Sammy's anal penetration wishes and fears, he spontaneously goes on to say, 'And that makes me think that I'm always shutting doors. I have to shut them or I get scared' (compare the dream in Session 116). He starts coughing, comes over towards my chair and splutters in my face. From there he goes on to talk about day-dreams that he has in the lavatory.

S. – When I'm sitting in the bathroom, I make most of my stories around the door. I pretend the door is a subway, and a train is just pulling out. Then the cross on the wall is a boat, but you can't get near it. It's always the same distance away.

Sammy constructs a boat with a sheet of paper and for the first time in weeks starts singing the Funeral March. He then talks of an old lady who used to be his baby-sitter in the States. It was she who taught him how to make paper boats.

S. – I wonder if she still remembers me, if she's not dead yet! (He starts hitting me and coughing all over me.)

J. M. – You really want to get rid of me today, Sammy. Perhaps you're afraid I shall not remember you.

Sammy laughs at the idea that he is coughing all over me in order to do away with me.

That evening, the Director of the Special School telephoned me. He had just seen Sammy and told me that Sammy was 'definitely schizophrenic' and that he felt that the school would be very suitable for his needs. He mentioned that during his interview Sammy kept rearranging the chairs in his toom, which had been moved by the Director. He had also asked Sammy to name three wishes, and Sammy had given the following responses: first, he wished for perfect health when he would be an adult; second, he wanted to be the most intelligent person in the world; and third, he wanted to be the most famous.

I said that I thought it was disturbing for Sammy to break off his analysis but he assured me that Sammy would continue to have psychotherapy in the Special School.

121st Session (Friday 14.5.55)

Sammy does a great deal of 'special talking' today. There is no trace of his recent reasonableness and closer apprehension of reality. He is visibly tense and anxious.

> S.–I saw the Director of the school yesterday. He's a lot better than you are. (Screams.) You have his penis and Dr Lebovici's too!

He then spends a long time discussing the metro and the problem it causes him when it does not pass the notice. He moves his chair closer to mine whilst he is talking, and suddenly shouts: 'Look out, this is my penis!' He rams his chair several times into mine, demands milk to drink, sets about hitting me, and at one moment kisses me in a very aggressive manner.

> J. M.–Perhaps you find me dangerous today, Sammy, because you are going back to America. You feel I'm abandoning you and sending you away.

Sammy then makes a number of drawings without coherent stories—a series of mountains and people trying to catch something. At the end of the session, he makes a great fuss about leaving: yelling, jumping around, and kicking, as he did in the old days.

> I feel he was trying in a confused way to express his need for contact. He is frightened by the coming separation and he still feels that I have the hidden magic he wants to possess.

Although he tries to build up his image of the Director, he immediately invokes my omnipotence—I am once more the devouring female who has stolen the male analysts' penises.

122nd Session (Monday 16.5.55)

Sammy arrives at the door with a policeman on each side holding his wrists! There was an open fair in the boulevard not far from my consulting-rooms and Sammy had arrived early in order to wander round there. The police picked him up, thinking that he was playing truant from school. Sammy refused to give his name, address, or any other details, except to say that he was American and that he had come to see a lady, whereupon the police accompanied him to my door. Sammy's little face is white and stiff with terror. I explain the situation to the police, who let him go, and then explain to Sammy the reason for his 'arrest'.

Sammy tells of the terrifying things he imagined were about to happen to him. His hands are black from touching the train; he smells them continually and talks excitedly about the view of the train seen from the top. He gives a great number of details rich in anal symbolism, concerning his delight in touching and smelling. I interpret the material for him in this way.

> S. – I like looking at the train at funny angles too. Do you ever look at your hindy?

He comes over and tries to rub the dirt on his hands all over me, telling me at the same time how much he likes me.

> J. M. – You seem to think that this is a way of love-making, and the sort of thing you imagine men and women might do with one another sexually.

This reference to intercourse leads Sammy to give many details about a peculiar noise the train makes as it screeches along the rails. He says, 'It's a very special noise and I'm afraid to imitate it.' After much drama over whether he may or not permit himself to make this noise, he reproduces one of the series of jerky squeaks and shouts, which closely resembles his 'special talking'. We again go over the anal-sexual meaning of these noises, and Sammy then gives further details about the metro at the station 'Etoile' where he can often enjoy the exciting spectacle of one train in the tunnel and one outside it. He is most excitable, and at the end of the session jumps on to my lap and makes a fuss about leaving. I talk to him again about the policeman, as representatives of paternal authority, and interpret his fear of leaving me in this connection.

123rd Session (Tuesday 17.5.55)

Throughout the session Sammy is disturbed and at times dissociated. He sings wild themes, pushes things over and occasionally hits out at me or punches my bottom. I tell him that he seems to be going back to some of his old ways of defending himself against anxiety. He feels I am deserting him because he is going back to America. All this makes him more angry with me. At one moment he asks for the old toys to play with again. When I point out his attempt to revert to his old anal defences, etc. he says: 'Oh, oh, I feel ashamed. It isn't progress I'm making!' He nevertheless picks up the toys, sings the Funeral March and suggests an aggressive game with Flicker and the Pink Boy.

S. – There are two leaders now. You'd better get a pencil to write.

I make no move to write and he does not insist on it in any way. He plays out a game where Flicker goes fart-fart and the Pink Boy does peepee in Flicker's belly.

At the end of the session, Sammy says: 'Oh, I'm sorry I did that silly game. Why did I do it? Is it very bad?'

> He is regressing in spite of his attempts not to do so. The visit with the Director of the Special School and the threat of leaving Paris have clearly precipitated this backward movement.

124th Session (Thursday 19.5.55)

The regression continues. Sammy begins the session shouting incoherently, singing snatches of Beethoven symphonies; then draws a series of wild, aimless scribbles covered with crosses and executed to the tune of the Funeral March. His behaviour is exactly like that in the early stages of his analysis. At one point he gets up and

203

starts running around the room, then rolling on the floor and giggling.

> S. – I don't think I have any more troubles, that's why I'm bored. What do you think?

I interpret his behaviour in much the same way as the 'special talking'. I point out to him his present resistance and the renewed hostility towards me, and the reasons for this. He slowly quietens down, and takes up questions about people's bottoms, attempting himself to find pathological reasons for this interest, until finally he is talking quite naturally once again. He shows great interest in his regressive behaviour of the last two sessions and the reasons for it. He follows this with a number of drawings of mountains and towards the end of the session talks about a new difficulty he has noticed in himself—his inability to concentrate on what he is doing.

> S. – When I think, it's as if I'm in another world. I don't know where I am any more or what I'm doing. It's a bit like that dream-feeling I used to have, but not as frightening.

He gives examples of his day-dreams, imagines that he is going to invent a drinking machine which he can take with him anywhere and which will supply many varied drinks, etc. He asks if this getting lost in his thoughts is a way of feeling protected from the world.

When we talked of its connections with his problems and the threatened departure from France, his 'special talking' reappears and continues until the end of the session.

> Although in this, as in the preceding session, Sammy reproduces the behaviour he had at the beginning, it is nevertheless relatively controlled. I think he is dramatising for me his need for the analysis. The 'special talking' helps to shut out his awareness of separation and re-establish a magical sexual union.

125th Session (Friday 20.5.55)

Sammy spends much of the session describing his need to arrange things. This need is felt as a pressing obligation. He tells me that in the waiting-room he always 'classifies' my magazines. At home, he constantly straightens the books on his book-shelves. He keeps the chairs in his room in special places and gets worried when they are moved. He frequently needs to shut all the doors and windows in different rooms. Sammy insists on an explanation because he recognises the absurdity of these acts as well as their compulsive quality.

J. M. – I suppose it all helps you to feel a bit safer. Perhaps if you have everything around you under control and nice and tidy, it makes you feel that the thoughts and feelings inside you are controlled too.

S. – You know, I don't day-dream very much now. Maybe that's why I tidy things up, and I never think of looking at the buildings these days to see what they're like. I guess they're getting on alright without my having to worry.

He starts talking again about his fascination with trains, but he talks of them as objects in themselves and not personified. He then comments on the fact that he has used no 'special talking' at all today. He makes a painting of 'the Jungfrau'.

S. – Why am I so interested in mountains these days?

I try to lead him out on his associations with mountains and particularly to the Jungfrau, thinking that he knows its English translation, but he shows no interest in following this up and I give no interpretation.

At the end of the session he is angry because the paint-box is dirty and he has not had time to clean it. His father comes for him today, and the moment Sammy sees him, he plunges into his 'special talking'. I note that the obsessional-type mechanisms which have been coming to the fore in the last few weeks are helping Sammy cope with traumatic and guilt-making emotional situations, and have partially replaced many of his earlier psychotic defences.

126th Session (Saturday 21.5.55)

Sammy seems to be 'back to normal' today, calmer and more reasonable. He examines carefully yesterday's painting of the Jungfrau, then does a painting of 'A Blizzard'. He studies this second painting closely, saying that it must mean something, because he feels so intensely interested in these Alps. Suddenly he shouts out: 'Dougie, I've got it! I have the meaning of it. These alps are breasts with all this blizzard coming out of them. And these are penises that I've drawn coming out of the side. And here is a bird coming to break off your penis—no, I mean your breast.'

He sets to, cleaning up the paints meticulously and with evident pleasure. He goes so far as to clean them with white paint and draws my attention to his carefulness in this respect.

> S.–Most people wouldn't even bother, you know. (As though struck by a sudden idea.) Oh dear, is it a trouble? It might be a trouble because I feel I *have* to do it. Why do I have to do it anyway?

I get the feeling that Sammy is cleaning or repairing me after the aggressive fantasy about breaking my breast-penis.

127th Session (Monday 23.5.55)

> S.–Last night I dreamed I was rising up in a lift and I saw life pass by through the grill.

He goes on to give fragmentary associations and does not accept my suggestion that he is retreating from life because he is anxious about threatened separation.

> S.–Oh, I might just as well talk to the wall as to you. Would that cure me?

128th Session (Tuesday 24.5.55)

Since Sammy's parents visited me last night, he asks a great number of questions today. He does not seek answers to his questions, but tries to estimate to what extent his parents are aware of the progress he recognises in himself. When Sammy comes to talk about the American school, he immediately begins 'special talking'. I show him once again that this is a way of expressing many hidden feelings, and encourage him to talk about his fear of having to leave Paris and me, to go to an unknown school. His flow of jerky speech calms down a little, and he asks if his parents mentioned the 'special talking' and whether they had talked of another difficulty—his inability to converse with two people at the same time. He also wonders whether his parents understand his 'day-dreams' problem.

S. – This still worries me a lot. If I find the buildings look sad because I'm going to have a good day, what does it mean, Dougie?

J. M. – It seems as though you think of yourself as somebody who has no right to have a happy day.

Sammy immediately starts to talk about the incident with the police the other day, then creeps into his chair and whispers: 'I'm a very, very bad boy.' He starts to whimper, then begins squealing and shouting, comes over to me and says; 'Quick, I want some milk.'

J. M. – As though you want something good inside you to soothe and control the feeling of being bad?

I remind him of his guilt about trains, and its associations with the police incident.

S. – Yes, yes, I know why I want it, but I'm still thirsty!

He summons Hélène and asks for a glass of milk and a glass of water. He drinks the milk, then makes a menacing movement as though he is going to throw the water, but finally sets the glass down.

S. – See, I *can* control myself. I'm not crazy.

He immediately begins to gallop round the room, hits out at my chair, seizes the wooden paper knife on my desk and begins to stab the chair with it. My interpretations go unheeded. He finally settles down to a certain extent, and does a drawing which he calls 'Blush' and which he says means 'being timid and happy at the same time'.

Towards the end of the session he is a little calmer and we are able to go over some of the elements of his troubled feelings during the last few sessions. He himself recognises that all his symptoms and behaviour problems have a meaning. Whereas in the past his regressive behaviour was used to ward off psychotic anxiety concerning annihilation and disintegration, he now seems to have at his disposal a number of neurotic defence mechanisms which he wishes to understand and to overcome. His 'Blush' picture introduces the idea of shame and self-criticism as does his remark, 'I can control myself—I'm not crazy'.

129th Session (Thursday 26.5.55)

Sammy is calm and almost grown-up in his manner. He says he is rather ashamed of himself because he hit a little girl at school. She had knocked off his glasses and this angered him. He tries to assess the extent of his 'badness' in taking this revenge.

S. – Yes, I seem to have to prove that I'm bad sometimes. I'm always afraid that God will punish me later. Gosh, I should have been dead long ago! You wouldn't understand because you're a Catholic. It's different for the Jews. And I did a second sin last night. I prayed to a little wooden cross, even though my father explained to me that this was not in the Jewish religion.

J. M. – Perhaps when you're afraid that God will punish you, it's a way of saying that you are afraid of your father.

S. – (In a very shocked voice.) Dougie, you don't believe in God?

He then goes on to describe a troubling experience the other day at the dinner table when there was a guest at home. (I wondered if this guest prefigured the coming visit of the Special School Director.)

S. – All the people suddenly went still. I was staring at the clock on the wall which looked funny and seemed to have stopped too. Everything got far off; I felt funny and afraid, and I tried to remember all the things we had talked about here, to help me. Then I had an idea that I didn't really believe in, but it stayed at the back of my head like a thought. I felt I ought to stay up late because my parents might do something very strange with the visitor. I tried to think about all the things you'd told me and I said to myself it was just a thought inside me, and nothing to do with the people outside. So after that, that trouble went away and it didn't seem to matter any more.

He continues to talk about his thinking difficulties, attempting to describe as accurately as possible what he feels.

S. – Well, it happens like this sometimes. Let's say I was thinking that I were dead. Well no, let's not take that one. Let's say, I may think of a word like 'Pamperyl' (trade-name of a fruit drink). Then I will see in front of me an island and then lots of smoke and a great black cloud. Well suddenly I look around me, and I can't remember at all what I've been thinking about, and I don't know how much time has gone by. Do others have this. What is it called?

J. M. – Well, we could call it a 'thinking trouble', and I think we can get to understand it a bit like the dream-feeling.

S. – Perhaps there are thinking troubles I don't even know about? I only have these two anyway!

He presses for information about other people's troubles, but accepts my intervention that his interest in others is a way of understanding his own problems.

S. – I just remembered a dream. I was at a fair and I fell into a 'thing'. It was a bit like our baby's bath. Then I saw an elevator with 'Chartres' written on it. There were lots of people around and they were all sick. (No doubt connected in Sammy's mind with the Special School.) I felt so sorry for them, but I suppose it's just because I worry so much about my own health. Then there was a long road and that's all.

(He goes on to talk about his friend Pierre at school, who acts all the time as though he does not hear a word anybody says.)

S. – I'm so afraid that it's what I'll have to put up with in the American school. I try to have conversations with Pierre, but it's no good, and I don't like Marie either because she always looks afraid. Then there's that little boy Antoine, who is Mme D's orphan child. I always wanted to see him beaten. I hoped she would get cross with him and I wanted to see his behind. Once she spanked him and I wanted to be him. I used to be afraid of being beaten by women with big, fat arms, but in another part of my head, I was calling out, 'Please keep on, oh please keep on.'

In the dream Sammy identifies with his little sister but in terms of a part-object (that which is exchanged between father and mother).

130th Session (Friday 27.5.55)

Sammy has brought along some fire-stones to show me. At one moment, he smells them and immediately asks for a drink of milk.

J. M. – To protect you from the smell?
S. – Hehe, yes, you're right. We can drop the milk!

He quickly starts to draw 'something exactly like a painting my father did. It's a driver in a bus and I have drawn it the way it looks from the inside.'

He goes on to talk about optical illusions with much delight, as though he is only just discovering the visual world and able to look at it without his veil of fantasy. His intense insistence on form and space perceptions gives me the impression that he may be using these visual observations as a way of controlling hallucinatory experiences too.

In a later session, he describes his tremendous difficulties in trying to draw or paint. His preoccupation with representational form is threatened at every moment by the invasion of fantasies connected with the people or objects he is trying to draw. The internal objects clamour for expression and interfere with the external world. Sammy then makes up some optical illusions for himself, and is very proud of them, saying he would like to take them to show his father. He asks a little anxiously if it matters that he is talking so much today. I limit myself to the interpretation that he perhaps feels safer in sharing these discoveries with his father rather than with me. He recalls then that some years ago, when he was a pupil for a short time, a boy in his class used to hit him and rub his legs up against him.

J. M. – How did you feel about that?

    S. – Oh, I wanted it, like as if I wanted a bit of him in me. I mean, when he was hurting me, it even felt good. Do you know what I mean?

J. M. – As if feeling the pain was like sharing in this boy's strength and getting something from him?

    S. – Yes, you said it just right!

> Since Sammy's oedipal development is still invaded with pre-genital drives I give no further interpretations; it is clear, however, that the 'woman with fat arms' whose beatings he desired when he was six contains a phallic representation (here represented by the boy friend who used to hit him).

131st Session (Tuesday 31.5.55)

A half-remembered dream in which Sammy receives a letter from Butch, then his problem concerning the 'disappearing thoughts' and other 'troubles' such as a fear that the walls around him are disintegrating, an idea that a book might suddenly eat its own pages or that words might turn into houses with children in them. These are all 'made-up troubles' and he is delighted that I have listened seriously to them.

> S. – I fooled you, didn't I?
> J. M. – It might be interesting to see why you chose these particular day-dreams to fool me with. (Are the disintegrating walls the analysis coming to an end, and consequent fear of internal damage of a devouring kind?)

Sammy immediately becomes very aggressive, jumps about and tries to hit me. I point out to him his apparent need to defend himself at moments when he feels me as dangerous, or rejecting.

> S. – But I don't pull your skirts up any more. You see, I do know how to control myself.
> J. M. – But sometimes it's as though you're afraid of being here peacefully with me.
> S. – Yes, I feel that something awful could happen. It's just that you have breasts *and* a vagina and I have only a penis, and — ugh — tell me (he stammers) there was a penis in that vagina wasn't there? (Screams.) You got my penis, I know you did! Tell me, tell me, I must know, you did take it, didn't you?
> J. M. – Perhaps it's important for you to believe that. The book which eats its own leaves is like my vagina wanting to eat up your penis, isn't it? If you imagine that I have taken the good things you possess you don't have to feel so worried about wanting all sorts of good things from me.

Sammy calms down quite suddenly.

> S. – Tell me, Dougie, why do I always worry about being in the biggest train?
> J. M. – Well, I suppose there are times when you feel small and helpless and you would like to be big, and feel as important as the big train. It's a bit like the way you felt the need to attack me today, as though you want to be big and strong like your father. (If Sammy renounces his penis he can only find potency through projective identification with a potent father or huge penis symbol.) But that becomes frightening because you see him as very strong and damaging too.

Sammy is now completely calm and quiet, and speaks very thoughtfully: 'I have some other worries, too, Dougie. There is this big worry about my insides. Is it the same thing, do you think? I wish I knew something I could say to myself when I feel a bit sick and I worry about dying. It helped so much to talk about that worry of my heart pains.' (The frightening internal relationships are modified and helped when externalised in the transference.)

Sammy goes on to give innumerable descriptions of bodily fears, as though there is little time left, and he must get them all out.

> I notice that whenever we talk of these fantasies of sexual exchange he almost invariably introjects aggressive images in which his 'insides' are attacked, and then his old hypochondriacal fears are reawakened immediately after.

132nd Session (Thursday 2.6.55)

Mothers' Day is approaching and Sammy describes the little gifts he is making. He debates for some time whether he shall make something for me or not, after a long soliloquy around the subject he slowly works up to an intense anger at the idea that I should get anything whatever from him, and ends up screaming that I shall have nothing at all and deserve to be punished.

S. – And anyway, you don't give me any presents, so just keep out of my way!

J. M. – All this talk about giving and taking makes you pretty angry. I expect you're still thinking like yesterday that I've taken all sorts of precious and valuable things away from you.

S. – Yes, and I want my lollipop back!

This lollipop is still in a drawer in my desk where Sammy left it some sessions ago. At the time, he was beside himself with anger because I didn't accept and eat this highly invested gift. He rushes to the drawer and pulls it out. At first, he is indignant to find that I have still not eaten it, but immediately afterwards is highly delighted and reassured to know that it still exists.

S. – I'm sure glad it's so safe but I wonder why you didn't take it last time when I said you were to eat it.

J. M. – You know I thought it was more important for us to understand what it really meant to give me this lollipop. If you remember, I felt at the time that you were insisting I must take it because you wanted to prevent me eating anything else of yours—your penis and all the other things that you value in yourself. But today you feel I have kept it nice and safe inside my drawer.

On the previous occasion, Sammy had been completely inaccessible to any discussion of this particular piece of acting out, but now he is very interested in the connection between the lollipop incident and his fantasies. However, as he continues to talk about it, his anxiety begins to mount. He becomes restless, throws one or two objects around the room, accompanied by a slow disintegration in his conversation. He is aware of this himself, stops suddenly and says he feels he is not making 'progress' in his analysis. I tell him that his fantasies are all starting to get outside him again, but that the more we can talk about them the more chance we have of understanding them and making them less frightening. Sammy immediately sits down and recalls a dream he had last night.

> S. – I dream I am in bed and a boy I once knew called Paul is there with me, and he does peepee in my bed. Then he disappears, and I hear him next door in the toilet. He makes 'ah-ah-ah' noises, and I can hear Mme Cor in there with him, helping him.

Sammy gives numerous spontaneous associations to the anal-urethral elements of the dream, mostly relating to his sister, and indicating considerable envy of her urethral and anal liberty and of all the attention she enjoys from Mme Cor on this account. I interpret his jealousy of his little sister, and his wish to exchange with Paul (a less dangerous object) all the exciting things that his little sister exchanges in connection with the nanny and his mother. This leads Sammy to floods of associations concerning his great friend Butch, which all express in thinly disguised form the possibility of sexual exchanges of this kind with Butch. I interpret his fantasy wish for masturbation games with Butch. He can furnish no associations whatever to the boy called Paul, who seems to have been a dream substitute for Butch and the little sister.

The session ends with a return to aggressive acting out towards me, no doubt connected with his concentrated interest in the analysis of his dream and subsequent feelings that I will forbid his double attempt to recuperate his own virility—first through a pre-genital exchange with a male figure, second by taking the privileged place of the little sister with the mother.

> Finding the lollipop-penis still intact helps Sammy to triumph over the frightening fantasy that if it has not been eaten he is still in danger of being devoured! In protesting against the absence of gifts from me Sammy sets up a vicious circle leading from the search for a warm relationship with the good maternal part-object to frustration experienced from it. It then becomes bad and stirs up fear and hostility. Sammy attempts to control these feelings; throughout his tragic and desperate struggle he is aware that the analysis has to some extent made this possible for him.

133rd Session (Friday 3.6.55)

Throughout the session Sammy reiterates: 'I don't have any more troubles; I don't need you any more.'

In between attempting to hit me and knocking the furniture around, he expresses considerable pleasure in the following ideas:

(i) that he has made a number of presents for his mother and that there will be nothing at all for me;

(ii) that it is wonderful to realise he no longer needs me for his troubles;

(iii) that he is getting on extremely well at school, which is further proof that he does not need my help.

Towards the end of the session I sum up the gist of his conversation and show him his complete denial of any need. I tell him that perhaps he is trying to reassure himself that I am not abandoning him by letting him go back to America; it is a way of abandoning me first. He then tells me that it is imperative that he jump on my stomach and makes many attempts to jump into my lap. I suggest that he is perhaps afraid that I have a little sister in my stomach who will get all my attention once he is gone. Maybe he even wants to get inside and become Dougie's baby.

134th Session (Saturday 4.6.55)

Sammy's behaviour is entirely different from yesterday's session— he is quiet, reasonable, and avid to understand his feelings.

S.–Things are pretty bad in our house at the moment. My father has the 'flu. Oh, I do hope he'll be well enough tonight to eat with me and my mother, because we have a lobster for dinner. And yesterday was not too good either. My sister was crying terribly when my mother and I arrived home. I went into my room and cried and cried. She had woken up at 5 o'clock this morning crying like that and I felt terrible. I said to myself: 'Don't be silly; it's alright. Don't exaggerate.' I don't know why I do it, talking to myself like that, and I wish I knew why it makes me cry so much.

J. M.–It looks as though you want to act exactly like your little sister. Perhaps it's a way of not having to get cross with her when she wakes you up with her crying. You're pretending to *be* her instead.

S.–I never told you how mad I used to get at her. I used to pretend to myself that I was sticking her whole head up with Scotch tape, and putting my hands over her mouth. I think I once did it really, too. (This is the first time Sammy has ever expressed a frankly aggressive feeling towards his sister.) I love to have her in my bed. Sometimes I put her head just there where my penis is and I make her suck it just like I was her mother. Once I put her hands on my chest and I pretended to myself I was feeding her. I really *was* her mother. But especially my penis—I want her to take it in her mouth just like a breast. Why do I want that, Dougie?

J. M.–It sounds as if you'd like to be very special and important just like your mother, and in this way you and your father would be the parents and Anne would be your baby. If you were the one who could feed her, you wouldn't need to have any of these jealous feelings about her and you also wouldn't have to be afraid of all the feelings that might bother you about your mother. You would really *be* your mother instead.

S.–That makes me think now of New Jersey being higher up than New York. Then the thought comes to me that I can manage not to be afraid of New Jersey. I don't know why I think of these things.

J. M.–You remember the time you were worried about my breasts being higher than your penis, as though you felt the breasts were very dangerous? Perhaps in the idea of feeding Anne with your penis there is the feeling that this way you would sort of have breasts too. Then you wouldn't worry so much

215

about losing your penis. It might seem like a safe way of having feelings in your penis.

S. – You know, I think that's right, oh, Dougie, I'm sure it is.

He goes on to talk again about the buildings looking cross if something nice is going to happen to him and this leads him to recall our earlier discussions of the way in which he throws his bad feelings outside of himself. From there, he talks of his bad and angry thoughts about his sister, and is suddenly surprised by the thought that perhaps he can have angry feelings without it's being dangerous.

S. – You know, Dougie, sometimes I imagine that I have to choose between my sister and myself getting killed. Or my mother and myself, or my father. It's really a terrible trouble. Mostly I think about it with my sister.

J. M. – Well, there must be some reason for you to make up this frightening idea. Maybe it's a sort of game you play — a way of getting rid of your angry feelings about your family and about Anne. You always thought you mustn't have such feelings. It's as though you say to yourself, 'I must not be angry with them so I'll make up a story in which one of them has to get killed.' But you feel so afraid of the angry thoughts that you imagine you might have to get killed yourself.

Sammy appears extremely relieved by this interpretation. He talks about a dozen other thoughts of a similar kind, but says that none of them made him feel so guilty and anxious as the fantasy of having to choose victims.

As he went out of the door with his mother, he said, 'I'm so happy today, I worked very well in my analysis.'

> In structures like Sammy's the interpretation of material such as his remarks about the height of the two cities (which it is inappropriate to call symbolic, since it is symbolic only in our eyes) leads to an alleviation of anxiety and to the production of new material. Here identification with the mother is completed by a fantasy of a baby which is nourished by father's penis.

135th Session (Monday 6.6.55)

Sammy is again reasonable and calm. He begins by telling me that he has lost his purse and is very bothered about it because it has 50 francs in it. He then mentions that he passed an adult patient on the stairs and discusses the effect that this has on him—his desire to know what this person's difficulties are, etc. He remarks that his father is now over the 'flu and asks if he may have a glass of milk: 'This time it isn't because I want to be sure that you will treat me like a good mother. I really am thirsty. I thought about it when I came in, but I didn't want to ask because I didn't want you to think that I was back on those old things again. You know at school today they gave me lettuce to eat and it made me choke. Mme Dupont told me that you can choke to death if you are weak. I was terrified. Really Dougie, I turned quite pale!

J. M.—Women will give you things that can kill you?

    S.—Oh but I don't *really* think so. You know, our baby is crying a lot more lately; the noise bothers me so much. Even my mother said she was tired of it, so you see it really is annoying. I used to have another kind of day-dream when she howled. I would think there was a man up in a corner of the room with a long thin knife and that he would swoop down and kill her. But even that didn't help. What would someone who had no troubles at all do when things bothered him like that? I mean somebody who understood perfectly and had listened carefully to his analysis?

I explain at length to Sammy the way in which he uses his day-dreams to cope with difficult reality situations, like trying to change the situation in fantasy or just running away from it, and show him that although this helps him to tolerate his feelings, it is not a very efficient defence. Sammy understands immediately the use he makes of day-dreams in this and other situations, and says that he sees that it is not too helpful, since it does not stop his sister crying. He starts to imagine other ways of dealing with such problems, and wonders whether he could not just go off and do something interesting for himself.

    S.—That makes me think of another trouble though. I often push little toy cars around and make noises like driving. I'm not thinking of anything special when I do it, but it's as though I'm driving it myself. I'm ashamed to tell you about it. It seems babyish. Is it alright to do that?

J. M.—It seems to me that you are just playing with the car as if you had a real one of your own.

S. – (Looking rather surprised and puzzled.) Is that playing? Yes, it must be. Is it a bad thing to do?

J. M. – You still think everything you like to do is bad.

S. – I don't really understand why I do it.

J. M. – All children like playing. It helps us to grow up, like practising to be an adult.

Sammy is astonished and reflects that perhaps he is becoming more like other children.

136th Session (Tuesday 7.6.55)

We spend most of the session on Sammy's thinking troubles. He says that the 'disappearing thoughts' trouble is occurring nearly every day now. He insists on several occasions that I help him to understand this phenomenon and asks if there is not something he can say to himself just to make the problem go away. We discuss it from the angle of defence: that it can be a means of running away from all the disturbing thoughts we have been analysing and that if he can find out what these thoughts mean he may not need to make them disappear.

137th Session (Thursday 9.6.55)

Antoine, Sammy's school friend, has very fat legs which fascinate Sammy. He stares at them for hours in spite of efforts to detach his gaze.

S. – Oh, his legs, his long round legs. I want to touch his legs so badly just like I always wanted to touch your bottom. (Just as the bottom included displacement from the breast, now the legs contain penis displacement ideas.) And there's another thing. His mother comes to collect him after school and she kisses him. I wish she would kiss me like that, but it's even more important about his legs. And there's another thing that happens to me now. I can't stop watching the plasterers who are working outside our house. They're working on the walls and I stare at them all afternoon. Is it a bad thing that I can't stop watching them? I want to see more and more of those men.

J. M. – Perhaps it's rather like Antoine's legs. You want to be part of
the things you stare at, and you feel that if you look at them
long enough you really possess them inside you. Perhaps it's a
way of feeling like a strong, whole kind of masculine person.
But I expect you feel it's bad, because you want to take something away from Antoine or from the plasterers.

S. – It makes me think of another worry I have about things
inside me. Sometimes I feel full of fart-fart gas, and I say to
myself I cannot keep it in, I have to let it out. I like letting it
out, but I think it's bad.

Since Sammy is currently expressing more and more freely
his homosexual wishes I refrain from interpreting, for the
time being, their oedipal context as well as the regressive anal
expression of his phallic wishes.

138th Session (Friday 10.6.55)

Sammy continues to be chatty and calm. He talks about painters
and paintings that he likes, much as though he were visiting a friend
and making conversation. He then mentions a visitor, a man who
often comes around to his home with his chest bare. This is a source
of fascination and of trouble to Sammy. He comments that male
chests are better than female ones, and then immediately takes up
yesterday's conversation about the plasterers. He looked at them for
a long time again this morning, and at school he also looked at
Antoine's legs and managed to touch them as though by accident.
While relating this incident, he becomes excited and describes his
feelings in a rapid stream of words.

S. – Oh, I would like so much to kiss and rub my head and my legs
and my penis and all of me right into all of him. And oh, and
all of me. Bit by bit inside him. And then he would not *be* any
more.

J. M. – As if you would like to eat him all up and get him into you
that way?

S. – Yes, but I want to go in his behind through the crack, right
up and get inside and eat him all the way up from there. Is
there any thought behind that?

J. M. – Well, wanting to get right inside him and wanting to eat him up at the same time sounds like the sort of things a baby wants from its mother. But so often you have this sort of feeling, not about your mother but about men or boys.

S. – Yes, that's right. I wonder why I don't have these feelings about women?

J. M. – Perhaps it might seem too dangerous to you. You remember that day-dream you had about breasts coming out and attacking you and making you loose your penis? It could be that you would be afraid of having these eating-up and getting-inside feelings towards women in case they might have the same ideas towards you. Someone with a penis might seem safer.

Sammy continues to elaborate the primitive mechanisms which lead to the formation of his homosexual fantasies. His vivid incorporation fantasy in which he will 'possess' Antoine from the inside throws light on the defensive value of projective fusion. It is interesting to see that anal penetration is here equated with oral aggression—rather like Jonah who fed on the inside of the whale who swallowed him. He who wishes to devour and incorporate can achieve this by being incorporated by his partner.

Sammy clearly wants to become Antoine to get the mother's kisses. No doubt his staring at the workmen is also an expression of phallic envy which at the oedipal level would be a desire for masculinity but for Sammy represents also a means of detaching himself from the dangerous aspects of the mother-imago. He feels guilty because of his oedipal wishes, but even more because of his wish for separate identity from the mother-figure which he can best achieve through a narcissistic identification with the males—Paul, Butch, Antoine, or the builders (including their reparative, constructive function.)

139th Session (Saturday 11.6.55)

Throughout this session Sammy behaves and talks almost like a normal child of his age. At the beginning of the session he announces that one of his teeth has just come out. He holds the tooth in his hand and asks if he might rinse out his mouth because it is bleeding. After a visit to the bathroom, he tells me that on his way back to the consulting-room he peeped into a corridor leading to the back of the apartment where he saw a number of children's paintings on the wall. (Paintings done by my own children.)

He then announces that he would like to leave his tooth with me. He pointedly avoids asking me to accept the tooth as a gift, but simply puts it in the drawer where the lollipop was formerly.

S.–I would really like to play some records here, but perhaps I shouldn't. After all, what would your husband say if he came in?

J. M.–You feel we would be doing something forbidden if we listened to music together and that my husband might be angry?

S.–Oh, you! You like your belly, that's what.

J. M.–Maybe it's you who likes my belly and wants to put something in it—like your tooth in my drawer. Perhaps it was an idea like that which made you afraid of what my husband would say.

Sammy smiles suddenly and says that he feels that after all there is nothing to worry about in listening to a record. He puts on a Brandenberg Concerto, then settles down to a long, adolescent-like conversation, in which he discusses the composers he prefers, with some appreciation of their compositions. He tells me he has made serious attempts to appreciate modern music, in particular Bartok and Stravinsky, but cannot get to like them. He is sorry about this because his father is very appreciative of modern music. He expresses a wish to learn to play the piano, and gives his opinion of flutes and recorders. From there he goes on to painters and paintings. He is critical of Rousseau and Seurat, but stresses his appreciation of Cimbué and Rembrandt. As with his musical tastes, he comments on his preference for classical painters and his inability to appreciate moderns. Abstract paintings and music are 'worrying', but he is making earnest attempts to understand his father's taste in music and art. At this point, he draws my attention to the fact that he is conversing and not listening to the record.

Now he talks about the guests who are expected that evening for dinner, in particular, the man already mentioned who leaves his shirt open. Sammy explores the probable reasons for this friend's aberration and becomes quite confused in his speculations.

S.–It bothers me. It reminds me of something troubling and I can't remember what.

J. M.–You know how often your interest in women is hidden behind an interest in a man. Might it be a way of hiding your interest in women's breasts, as well as wanting to get close to the man?

S.–Oh, that. I'm not sure. Anyway if I'm allowed to stay up late tonight it's because I like the women *so much*. But about our friend showing his bare chest. Please tell me, Dougie, what would a person who had no troubles at all do if his friend left his shirt open?

I ask Sammy what in fact he does do in such circumstances. Sammy replies that he makes a great number of remarks about it to the friend in question (the parents have already reported that the friend is highly embarrassed by Sammy's overwhelming interest in his chest). Sammy is vaguely aware that the friend becomes upset and accepts with interest my intervention that people do not usually like personal remarks of this kind and would not necessarily understand how anxious Sammy is feeling. He then plunges into a discussion about adults who might need analysis and passes from there to wondering if other children need to do drawings and tell stories the way he used to do when he came to see me. He says he is making progress in his analysis because he no longer needs to do drawings in order to feel at ease here. He asks if it is essential to have troubles to talk about.

J. M.–Everything that you talk about is interesting in analysis. It doesn't have to be a trouble. Today you have told me your ideas about all kinds of things as though you felt like having a friendly talk rather than being a patient with 'troubles', and perhaps also it's a way of proving that you can be like this with me without feeling that you're in any danger.

S.–Maybe I wanted to have music today so as not to be a patient! I've got over wanting to bring my own records in here to play. I have a sort of trouble about the 7th Symphony though. I don't want to play it at home any more. It reminds me of all the fart-fart and the death things and all those sad things in the beginning of my analysis. I never want to go back to those things, Dougie. The 13th Concerto is very sad, too. It reminds me of the time when there was hardly anything in my life that I liked. I never listened to any music except Beethoven and I always wanted to be alone. I was very sad always. But this time I *really* don't want to hear the 7th Symphony at home. It's not something like a trouble. It's not because I think it's bad or anything and still want to do it. I just don't want to listen to it.

The end of the session coincides with the end of the record.

S.-I think the music helped me to talk. It's easier with music going on.

I felt throughout this session that words had regained their communicative value for Sammy and were not at any moment invaded by primitive impulses or their defences. He has less need, at least for short periods, to project frightening impulses on to me. The control and maturity Sammy demonstrates here was almost certainly mobilised by the coming dinner during which he will again be confronted with the 'friend with the bare chest'. He is desperately trying to be more grown-up both to control his rising anxiety and because of his growing awareness of the critical attitudes of those around him when his social behaviour is bizarre or embarrassing.

140th Session (Monday 13.6.55)

Sammy has received a letter from Butch. He is terribly excited about it, but dallies with the idea of making Butch wait several months for a reply. In this way, he says, he hopes to avoid the pain of having to wait for a letter himself and envisages punishing Butch at the same time. He goes on to speak of a little girl friend he once had, called Jenny.

S.-It was in a special school I once went to. I want to marry her. Is that alright? You know, she's a bit like me. She's very quiet and not like other people. Maybe she's awfully afraid of boys, but not of me. She's so understandable and kind. I really think I could marry her and have children. I think I want to, and I'm sure she would like it. I don't think it's bad, is it?

Sammy gives many details of his fantasy of marrying Jenny, but outlines all these projects in a calm, detached voice and shows none

223

of his usual excitement. He gets round to talking about Butch and the tone suddenly changes. He shouts: 'But my friend Butch, oh that Butch!' He begins to jump excitedly on to his chair, then starts to push his chair aggressively into mine.

J. M. – You are much more excited talking about Butch than about Jenny.

Sammy comes over to my chair with his fists clenched and a gleam of hatred in his eyes.

S. – Yes, I love you! Oh, I love you! (said in a tone of intense hostility).

He jumps on to the arm of my chair, begins kissing me, and suddenly turns to bite me. Meanwhile, he reiterates that he loves me.

J. M. – Why do you think you want to bite me, suddenly?
S. – But I really do love you. I don't know why I bite. I say, did you see in the papers today about all those people that got killed? (referring to news of a serious local train crash).
J. M. – You talk about loving, but I think it immediately frightens you into thinking about people who get killed!

Sammy is meanwhile manœuvring his chair still closer to mine, saying, 'I want to be higher; I must; I'll get to you, you'll see!' Without warning he jumps on to my lap and murmers: 'Mmmm, mmmum, mmumm, mother and son, mother and son.'

J. M. – Perhaps this is the way you want to be with your mother, with loving and hating all mixed up.

Sammy springs off my lap and begins gambolling in and out around the chairs.

S. – What am I thinking about now?
J. M. – Well, you tell me!
S. – In the front of my head I'm just playing, but in the back of my head I'm thinking that you have bosoms! I want to cut your hindy off, that's what! Have I got troubles today? Am I better?

I pointed out the resurgence of his feeling that I am dangerous to him, particularly when he talks about loving me. At that, he settles down to a long conversation about whether I would continue to see him if his mother didn't pay for his sessions. He reverts to trying to bite me, making references to biting bosoms, and without a break takes up again his theme of the friend who leaves his chest bare.

J. M. – Perhaps you feel the man will protect you against the bosoms that bite.

S. – You know, it makes me think of my mother's breasts. I'll never touch them again.

He makes a great fuss about leaving at the end of the session, and going out tries to hit me in the stomach, saying, 'I love your belly.' His mother is a few minutes late and he has to wait in the waiting-room. He writes a message which I find later on a piece of drawing paper. 'Help me with my troubles, Dougie, please.'

> Sammy mentions his eventual marriage with a little girl whom he feels, like himself, to be isolated in a hostile world. He is attracted to her, owing to the narcissistic reassurance which her difficulties provide for him, but his sexual excitement makes him turn to Butch instead. He feels obliged defensively to state that the little girl is the object of his affections.
>
> When he acts out in the transference, overwhelmed by the excitement aroused by drives which he cannot control, he is not attacking a woman or a man, so much as a combined mother-father figure. At this moment the sexual and aggressive drives are merged. Love and death have exactly the same significance, and love leads to death. Nothing could be more eloquent than the moment when Sammy, fighting to control these impulses, takes refuge on his analyst's knees and murmurs several times, 'Mother and son'.
>
> Like all psychotic children, his awareness of his most deep-seated problems leads him to dissociate what is going on in the front of his head (his play) from what is going on at the back (he is thinking that Dougie has bosoms).
>
> The analytic situation is complicated by the fact that Sammy knows he will soon have to leave. This no doubt explains why he needs to reassure himself that I would willingly look after him without payment, and why he leaves the sad little request in the waiting-room at the end of the session.

141st Session (Tuesday 14.6.55)

Sammy is aggressive and difficult. He talks frequently of wanting to jump on my stomach 'to get rid of all the sons you have there' and at another stage 'because you have eaten my penis off'.

I link this material and its fantasies with the anticipated rejection and also his slowly developing day-dreams about Butch.

> S.—I think it's about Butch that is most important. You see, at the back of my head I have the idea that you have Butch's penis in there, and when I see him, it'll be so awful, he won't have a penis any more.

I remind him that he has already had the idea that his mother did not want him to be too attached to Butch, and now maybe he thinks that I want to have Butch and his penis for myself. Perhaps we can get to understand his own feelings about Butch's penis.

> S.—Don't talk about Butch, Dougie. Don't, don't!

Sammy is not expressing a delusional idea when he claims I have Butch's penis inside me. He is play-acting but frightened nevertheless. His fear of the separation is felt as a castration and arouses hostility and guilt which he projects on to me. He senses, too, the aggression contained in his homosexual desires towards Butch and thus he projects on to me his desire to possess Butch's penis.

142nd Session (Thursday 16.6.55)

Sammy again exhibits enormous excitement over Butch. There is more than the usual amount of jumping up and down, giggling and squiggling around. He says he would rather not talk about it at all because by now he is terrified of the whole idea of ever seeing Butch again. From there he goes on to talk of all the dangers which lie around him every day. His terror of cars in the street, of strange people, of dogs, of anything that moves.

> S.—I spend all my time having frights about things. Why is that, Dougie? Oh but one thing is better—about my sister. I'm beginning to like her better. I don't need to have day-dreams when she cries now. She should be smacked, though. You know, I think the French method for children is better. They smack their children all the time.

226

From this settling of the sibling question, Sammy passes to thinking about my other patients. He would like to hear 'that they are very, very sick', and would be pleased to know that I get very angry with them. He would also like to know the reasons for which I might get angry with them. In and around this talk, he keeps remarking that he is making brave attempts to avoid the subject of Butch. He tells me this so often that I tell him my impression is that he wants me to make him talk about Butch. In addition, he keeps prefacing the Butch remarks with inciting asides like: 'What's your trouble today?'

143rd Session (Friday 17.6.55)

S. – Well, what's your trouble today?

He commences his crazy dancing and jumping, which is now automatically associated with thoughts about Butch, so today I call it 'The Butch Dance'. This 'dance' is accompanied by intermittent outbursts of aggression, sudden threats and menacing gestures.

S. – Oh that Butch, that Butch, whatever shall I do! I'll see him there in New York, (oh, oh, haha, etc., for about five minutes).

He then moves away from his favourite preoccupation to talk about his two goldfish.

S. – I bought two because I wanted to see them together. I bought them with my own money. Alone I bought them, see. *I don't need you.*

He is very pleased with this assertion, continues for some time on the same theme and accompanies this wish with movements of anger at moments when he remembers that it is not true.

S. – I hate you because I have to take just so much from you! (He pushes his chair near to mine.)
S. – And now I have a trouble. I have to write a letter on Sunday — to Butch! (He begins again the characteristic dance and jump routine.)
J. M. – There's the Butch Dance again, Sammy. You're doing all this instead of saying out your feelings about Butch.

S. –No, no!! (He subsides into his chair.) Yes, you're right. (For one moment, he seems completely calm.) But Dougie, what is going to happen when I see him? Ohohoh, hahahha. (He starts off again on his mad, excited dance.)

J. M. –You seem even too afraid to think about what you want to do with Butch.

S. –Well, it starts like this. I'm going towards him and then — (he breaks off abruptly). You know, the other day I was in the bath-tub and I soaped myself all over, and did my feet and legs, etc. etc.

He continues with a long story of his soaping and scrubbing rituals. When I pointed out that these might be associated with thoughts about Butch, he denies that he has ever made any day-dreams about him, but adds that the dreams about Butch never get finished as though he cannot concentrate on them.

J. M. –It seems you're afraid of your love feelings for Butch.

S. –Yes, I am, but I'm also afraid he will love me too. Dougie, just imagine, perhaps he'll even want to kiss me!

He repeats once more what he has often stressed, that in this friendship it was always Butch who kissed him much more. This time he tells of an episode when they were on the train together and they pushed their heads into each other's bellies. He concludes that his fears of the anticipated meeting are well-founded. He is afraid that at the moment of meeting Butch, 'he may faint or perhaps vomit, or have a pain'. He seems so contorted with anxiety that I explain to him that these different fantasy reactions are a defence against feeling too acutely his excitement over Butch; that what he *imagines* is the important thing to understand. This is what frightens him—not Butch.

Sammy continues to discuss his terror until the end of the session. At one moment, while talking of his fear of Butch, he leans forward and kisses me on the cheek, hitting me at the same time. I link his conflicting attitude to me to his excited and terrifying feelings for Butch. He keeps asking me to do something about his panic before the dreaded moment of meeting arrives, but at the same time is unable to follow on from any of my interventions. When I announce the end of the session, he taps me in the stomach and says, 'I love your belly!'

The increasing cathexis of Butch is obvious. He becomes a refuge in face of the impending separation and also a defence against oedipal and preoedipal aspects of the transference. I am in doubt about interpreting his homosexual feelings in their purely defensive aspect, since I sense his need to express more freely the partial drives involved.

144th Session (Saturday 18.6.55)

Sammy begins squeaking and dancing around, then summons Hélène to bring him a glass of water. He stands behind my chair tilting the glass slightly as though he would like to throw its contents over me. The fact that he has asked for water is by now almost synonymous with aggressive feeling in Sammy. When he wants to be soothed and to quieten feelings of anxiety, he almost invariably demands milk.

J. M. – Perhaps you're angry because yesterday I encouraged you to face your feelings about Butch?

Sammy continuous to gaze at me, making little noises to hold my attention. Meanwhile, he is covertly letting water trickle out of the glass on to the carpet.

J. M. – Is this a way of showing me, rather than telling me, what you feel about Butch? Like a little boy who wants to make peepee, as you once told me?

Sammy hastily sets the glass down, and pulls his chair up closer to mine.

S. – Now, what is it I want to say about Butch?
J. M. – Supposing you tell me.
S. – It always starts like this. When I arrive he will be there at the airport and we'll go together in the bus. . . . Then he'll take my hand. You know, I was in a bus once in Italy . . .

He goes off into general and lengthy descriptions of this holiday with his parents. Although the Butch longings are clearly connected with his father I leave this aside for the moment.

J. M. – I see what you mean about not being able to finish a day-dream connected with Butch.
S. – Oh! Oh dear, it's frightening, but I'll try again. Well, I get to the airport, then this Butch, ah, ah, he will kiss me ohohohoh.

Then I will say something to him. I'll say very crossly, 'Now are you satisfied?' If he says yes I'll be very, very happy. If not, ah, ah, ah (he squirms around as though in pain), I shall find an island where no one ever had any troubles, and a place where I would have some friends. Not too much friends. And they would be friends I don't love too much, and they'd all feel like that too. Look, I want to draw my island. Now, my family would be here and perhaps you'd be there; then here's my house with swing doors to it that people could not get into, just in case Butch ever came, and all around the island there would be these big mountains. (He goes on for some time protecting his island in this way.)

J. M. – So in this day-dream, you are running away to an island to protect yourself from the frightening and exciting feelings.

S. – (Looking literally astonished.) But Dougie, how ever did I get on to all this about the island? Where did I break off? I must try and get back to it. Well, I got to the airport—oh dear, I don't know what to do if he wants to kiss me. I'll look at my parents to see what I should do. Oh hell, I don't want to go to America! I'll just tell my parents I'm not interested in seeing Butch any more and I want to go and live in some other country. I know, I'll live all my life somewhere else. Oh, I forgot to tell you. There's trouble at my place. I did a painting this morning for my sister. My father liked it very much, so afterwards I was allowed to have her in my bed. Oh, oh, oh. (He groans and jumps up and down in his chair.)

J. M. – You know, Sammy, part of the feeling which frightens you so much about Butch has to do with feelings about your family, like the way you get excited and frightened when your father is pleased with you, and then the things you would like to do with your sister.

S. – Oh, Dougie, what'll I do? This Butch thing is bad, yet I can't tell you any more, I really can't!

J. M. – Perhaps you're concerned about what I would think?

S. – Oh, no. This is funny. I'm not at all afraid of what you'd say, and I think you could help me, but something in me won't let me say it. I can't, I can't. I don't even know how to say it. I just want to go and live in another country!

J. M. – You know that you can't run away from yourself just by going to live in another country.

230

S. – But Butch wouldn't be there, and it'll never happen again like
that, never.

J. M. – I think you would still feel things about people and *want* to do
so, in any country in the world.

S. – Well then, I'll go off the world!

He takes up a pencil and begins to draw his planet, enlarging
meanwhile on its descriptive details and its inaccessibility.

J. M. – These feelings must be very frightening for you Sammy, but I
think we can get round to talking about them. You remember
how difficult it used to be for you to talk about the fart-fart
and the funny thoughts?

S. – Yes, but that was different. Somehow I always knew I was
allowed to have these feelings. I couldn't say them to you
because I didn't know you then.

J. M. – And this time you are even more afraid so that in a way they
are stronger and more important feelings.

S. – I wish I were dead! (He takes up a pencil and draws his
corpse.) There, I've turned into stone. I'd like that. Stones
have no feelings, do they?

J. M. – I think you do turn yourself into stone in a way when you get
too scared of yourself. It's a bit like the dream-feeling that
frightened you so much. It's a way of trying not to feel
anything.

S. – Dougie, I must try and say out the whole thing about Butch.
Shall I try now? I think it would be a big progress.

Whereupon he develops a long day-dream about his first day with
his friend. He hesitates for some time about whether to have his
parents there or not. They meet at the airport, they kiss, they hold
hands briefly. Butch's mother sends them out to play and they walk
down the road together. They wander through the park telling each
other stories of what they've been doing and funny things they have
heard. Then they return and have tea.

S. – There! Are you pleased with me?

J. M. – Did it seem very terrible to tell?

S. – Yes, it did, but I did it! And I did say a lot—I didn't think I
could!

Sammy's homosexual fantasies have now attracted to them
all the guilt originally attached to his earlier anal excitements.

231

Any anticipation of desire is inevitably painful since Sammy is incapable of imagining any fulfilment or comfort, except in a state resembling death—the stone feeling.

145th Session (Monday 20.6.55)

S.–I wrote to Butch last night so now it's over. I'm imagining he might send me a letter back. (His voice drops to a whisper.) And love and kisses ohohoh!

He goes into a long pantomime, jumping up and down, squeaking and dancing, then sits down in his chair and makes the following series of drawings:

1. A barrier which he says is a fence between himself and his troubles.
2. Butch kissing him and Sammy saying 'No, no.'
   (S.–But it isn't Butch really. It's someone else who's going to kiss me and take all my troubles away. I wish it were Butch!)
3. Butch putting his hands on Sammy's face and Sammy smiling.
4. Sammy dead and Butch crying.

While doing these drawings, Sammy makes frequent reference to my belly, to his loving it and the need to hit it. He also recounts a womb-like fantasy he made in the bath. 'I was an island keeping myself safe out of the water, but the idea at the back of my head is that the water was Butch.' Towards the end of the session he tells me that there never was such a person as Butch; that photograph he once showed me was just a boy he hardly knew called Albert.

S.–You see, the whole thing is just a day-dream. I made it all up, but it's true that all my life I *wanted* a friend just like Butch.

J. M.–This looks like another way of getting rid of the Butch-trouble. Instead of making yourself dead, you are now making Butch the one who doesn't exist.

S.–Oh no, oh no! You're wrong—Butch is all made up, the whole idea! There isn't *any* Butch!!

146th Session (Tuesday 21.6.55)

Again the talk is all about Butch, but throughout his recital Sammy is constantly seeking physical contact with me. This time I bring some of the Butch material into the transference.

J. M. – It seems that you would like to do with me many of the things you dream of doing with Butch?

Sammy goes on unabated with his rough 'love-making' and attempts to hit me in the stomach.

J. M. – It seems as though you want to be very close to me and at the same time that you are really afraid of my belly. I wonder whether it's even easier to make up day-dreams about Butch than to talk about your feelings for me and the things that bother you.

In an attempt to deal with his homosexual wishes Sammy then does a drawing in which both he and Butch are dead.

S. – I'm so afraid. It'll all excite me too much! I just won't be able to go on living. I can't even do paintings the way I want to. One day I saw some paintings in your corridor—they aren't a bit like my paintings. Those are happy children without worries. When I draw it's different. I'm always worried about how it looks because it always *means* something. Like today I did some trees with the leaves folded all in around like that. (He gestures with his hands.) It had to be like that because it was Antoine's legs. I worked and worked and couldn't get the shape right. I wish I could draw ordinary things like other children.

Antoine is the boy about whom Sammy developed his fantasies of anal penetration (in Session 138). He has so few resources for dealing with his drives and they invade his desperate attempts to contain them in sublimated activity.

147th Session (Thursday 23.6.55)

Sammy is less agitated today, but immediately becomes aggressive and wants to hit me in the stomach whenever he talks about Butch. I point out his need to attack and punch me whenever he is faced with these feelings. Finally, he says he would like to draw a picture of what he really wants from Butch. The drawing is somewhat reminiscent of a mother and child portrait. Sammy writes under it, 'A picture of Butch holding me on his heart'. I ask him if he doesn't

233

think it rather like a mother and child and remind him of the many occasions when he has preferred to talk about Butch or some other masculine figure when he is really thinking about ideas connected with women. Sammy then notices that the picture of Butch has no body, only a head and chest. 'There now, I've put in their bottoms, just to show I'm not afraid, and here's their penises, and their BMs falling out. See, I can draw anything.'

He goes on to talk of the friend who bares his chest, and says he often thinks 'of cutting it up and eating bits of it'.

J. M. – It really sounds as if you want to love in the only way a baby can love it's mother, by eating her up. Perhaps that makes you afraid that women will be dangerous to you because of this feeling, so you would prefer to have these eating ideas about Butch or the grown-up friend.

S. – Oh, well then I can just go and bite my mother.

J. M. – Except that you're no longer a baby.

S. – Well, yes, I'm thinking about that, and about something else *too*. That time when I put my head on Butch's chest, it wasn't as nice as I thought it'd be, and I once touched my friend's bare chest; it wasn't so good; I touched Antoine's legs, too — that was wonderful, but not so wonderful as I thought either. I expect it'd be just the same with my mother.

Sammy is most enthusiastic about this discussion, and says that he has really understood something new.

S. – But Dougie, this is awfully important! You know, I now understand what it's all about, this analysis. I'm so lucky to have an anlyst. Some children can't have one, but Antoine and Pierre and Pascale wouldn't even enderstand what it's all about. How is it I understand that? They'd never understand. They would think you just go and talk about yourself to someone, but they wouldn't know it would be like this.

The mechanism which enables Sammy to escape from his primitive impulses to homosexual wishes (which are at first used a defence but soon become as guilt-ridden as the primitive impulses they are replacing) leads to a complex situation. The interpretation that the drives directed towards the mother are displaced is a constructive one. We can see that hidden behind Sammy's apparent homosexuality, there is the longing to recover a happiness which he has never found with his mother, and that it seems to him less dangerous to seek this happiness with men whose 'chests' when incorporated do not contain such dangerous objects as those imagined to be inside the mother. Sammy's reply to this interpretation is extremely interesting: 'I have only to go and bite my mother.' When older children in the course of a long analysis express such primitive fantasies, they usually bring day-dreams such as drinking milk, being fed at the breast again, etc., but Sammy's fantasy is about *biting* his mother.

The disillusionment he describes, in each of the oral relationships he imagines with substitute objects, is illuminating as well as tragic, since Sammy still needs to imagine that he would experience the same disillusionment with his mother. It is probable that Sammy was also conscious of disillusionment about the analysis and that he was preparing himself by taking in the analyst as a good object, when he spoke with enthusiasm of his good fortune in having an analyst.

148th Session (Friday 24.6.55)

Sammy pulls his chair close up to mine and for the first time in months asks if I have written down anything about yesterday's session. When I ask him what things interest him about the session, he goes on to day-dreams of Butch, accompanied by the same kinds of fantasies. He then draws a map showing himself and Butch walking off in the opposite directions. Meanwhile, he keeps leaning over to pinch my arms. I interpret these attacks in the light of the Butch fantasies and as an expression of his excitement. 'I love you', he says through clenched teeth. Claiming that he is tired, he then goes and lies on the divan, but immediately afterwards starts jumping up and down madly.

J. M. – You seem to be doing lots of things today instead of saying what you feel.

Sammy then begins playing with his feet and making little cooing and crying noises like a baby. He replies that it cannot be baby-like, because his little sister does not do it. He comes back to his chair and repeats in a hoarse, fierce voice, 'I love you', as though he really meant to say, 'I would love to kill you'.

J. M. – It seems to me, Sammy, that with all these angry thoughts of loving, you are afraid of feeling happy and loving when you are here with me, and perhaps when you are playing at being the baby this has something to do with what we were talking about yesterday. You would like to feel close and comforted like a baby, but at the same time this makes you angry, because you want much more than that.

149th Session (Saturday 25.6.55)

Sammy is still somewhat aggressive, but much calmer today. He talks a lot about his admiration for his body and describes how he loves watching his limbs when he is swimming and how much he admires the construction of his arms and hands. He says he finds himself very handsome and is sometimes fascinated with his body for hours after he has been swimming. We discuss his reassuring appreciation of the handsomeness of his body, as a way of feeling that he is whole and alright, but at the same time as something he can love when he is frightened of loving other people, since this is often so full of danger for him. This brings him back to talking of Butch, and his terror of what will happen when they meet again.

I point out to him the narcissistic aspect of his interest in Butch, whose body is like his, and his need to stick at this stage of reassurance because of all the fears he has towards the female sex.

150th Session (Monday 27.6.55)

Sammy asks innumerable questions about my family and becomes very angry at not getting detailed answers. I ask him whether this intense interest is associated with the fact that the summer holidays are starting in another week, and he will not be seeing me for some weeks.

He pushes his chair close to mine, then makes two drawings, one of himself and one of Butch. He tears Butch's picture to shreds, asks for matches to burn it up, and when he does not receive these, throws the fragments of Butch's portrait out of the window. He then places his own portrait on the mantelpiece. This done, he immediately comes back and hits me, shouting, 'Oh, that Butch!'

J. M. – You know, Sammy, it's really me you're angry with. You won't be seeing me for some time during the summer holidays, and in two months you have to leave altogether. I guess you feel it's all my fault. Although you have just thrown Butch out of the window, you perhaps feel that it is better to love Butch than Dougie, who leaves you all alone.

S. – Yeah, I love you!

He takes a long wooden paper knife which is lying on my desk and plays out a game of cutting off my head with it. He then passes to various other mimed aggressions, resembling closely the aggressive fantasies towards Butch. From time to time he mutters angrily: 'I want to kiss you', 'I love you' or 'I want to kill you' as though killing were the most satisfactory way of loving.

> The narcissistic defences which were in evidence for two or three sessions again pervade this session; for the privilege of having his portrait on the mantelpiece Sammy is even willing to destroy symbolically his homosexual bond with Butch. But at the same time he feels that I forbid his homosexual attachment.

151st Session (Tuesday 28.6.55)

Sammy is very chatty today and on the whole fairly peaceable. He brings two dreams: in the first, I am very cross and growl at him for arriving late. In the second I come to his house and tell him in an angry voice that 9 o'clock is too late for his bed-time. Sammy goes on to the spontaneous association that his father tells him he goes to bed too late and on one occasion had added that he was sure I would not approve of his staying up so late.

J. M. – It seems you might like me to growl at you and to be more like your father.

S. – Oh yes, I'd like that.

His obvious need to make me into a supportive superego figure leads him to face his feelings about Butch. He passes immediately to making a series of drawings intended to clarify this problem.

237

S. – That Butch gets on my nerves. I can feel him like as if he was sticking to me. Just like Scotch tape. I can't get him off my back. (This is like a negative version of Butch as water surrounding the Island-Sammy.)

152nd Session (Thursday 30.6.55)

Sammy goes on with his aggressive love declarations: 'I want to kiss you, and I want to thump you in the belly.' He tells a dream: 'I was walking along in a funny, loopy sort of way when I came to a flat just like ours. I found a big cave in the wall and I climbed right inside it.'

He continues immediately with the Butch fantasies, showing a great deal of pseudo-aggressive feeling against Butch and comes round to saying that he understands that all this hatred towards Butch is just to protect him from his positive feelings. It is frightening him less now, but yesterday for a short while he became so frightened of all his excitement that he tried to have the 'stone feeling' or the 'dream feeling' of depersonalisation once again, but it did not come back.

S. – I don't want to have any feelings about anyone. I don't need any feelings and I'm happier without them!

153rd Session (Friday 1.7.55)

Sammy spends the first fifteen minutes squeaking, rolling his eyes, dancing about and talking of Butch. He draws another series of Butch stories, complaining intermittently that Butch gets on his nerves or sticks to him. Later in the session, he says I get on his nerves and, as with Butch, while trying to explain the things I do to worry him, he makes slips of the tongue and talks of the things he wants to do to me. For example, 'Now just you get away, I want to kiss your hindy.' To escape from these ideas, he again gets back to talking of Butch. He is becoming more aware of the extent to which his fears of what Butch will do are his own fantasy wishes, and that these can be accepted as such and understood.

We discuss at length the fact that after tomorrow we will each be going on our summer holidays.

Sammy explains once more how Butch gets on his nerves. He writes all these statements down, then ties the papers together and gives them to me as though they were a present. He stresses that this packet must be hidden from his mother. After this, he says: 'Let's play husbands and wives.' Whereupon he jumps towards my chair, tries to hit me and makes determined attempts to bite me.

J. M. – Is this what you think husbands and wives do together?
S. – Well, only at the back of my head, but at the front of my head I know it isn't like that.

He goes on to talk about Butch intermingled with ideas of exciting and aggressive attacks upon me, confirming my feeling that behind all his terror about Butch, ideas of aggressive intercourse are coming closer to the surface.

> His desire to make me a gift of the Butch stories has at least two significant meanings: first he wants to leave all his troubling anxiety behind with me; at the same time he is leaving an important part of his libido. He still fears that women will forbid his homosexual wishes and thus block the way to masculine identification. (Mother must not know that he wants to get closer to father.) Having said this, however, he then acts out an oedipal wish in which he is my husband.

SUMMER HOLIDAYS   July–August 1955

During the holidays I did not see Sammy for seven weeks, but he kept in touch with me by a series of letters which are reproduced here in full. I answerd each of these but did not keep copies of my letters.

First letter — undated

Dear Dugie,
     I am very glad to be writing to you. Are you alright. I am very happy to tell you that I have lots of friends here. I have a boy friend and his name is Paul, and he is a very plezent boy and on Sundays I dance with lovely girls and I make L O V E with my mother. Very sad L O V E. I am very happy.

Lots of love, Sammy

239

I love my mother more than Butch. Ho ha ha. I will tell you the trooth. That you were rite I like to kiss my mother better than to kiss Butch. He gets on my nerves more and more and more. Bad bad Butch getting on my nerves and kisses me. I am glad to be far from very far from BAD BUTCH. I love my mother, just love. I love my mother more than Butch. Caca. I am mad.

Sammy

On the outside of the envelope was written 'bad letter' and on the inside flap 'bad Butch, good Sammy'.

Second letter—26 July 1955

Dear Dugie,

Your letter excited me so much that when I looked at the back of it to see who it was from I took a long time to open it. Then I must I will open it and read it and when I read it, it hurifide me to see the word Butch in it. Then it was so exciting that I was just about to tear your letter up to BITS. But I didn't du so because I would be very unhappy if I tore your letter boohoohoo.

Your letter got to my hotel just on time when I was beginning to worry a bit. And sometimes I all of a sudden worry about my helf, (health) for no reason at all. Then I think about Butch a bit and that calms me down. I am getting a looss tooth but I am not sure. It just wobels a bit. Sorry to interrupt the conversation about Butch but he just gets on my nerves a little too much. I should hope that when I get back to New York I will not worry Butch so much as I am now, because he just gets on my nerves MORE AND MORE EVERY DAY. Very TROO. But please Dugie don't tell me that I am afraid of my own fealings because I KNOW IT. I am much laiss worries about the American school business. By the way, you don't have to tell me that when I see Butch is bad that I am afraid of my own fealings about me, because you have said it about a 100 times, and also I don't lose my memory so fast, if you don't mind. By the way, I have this boy who left the hotel for a few days and I thought that he would never come back but he did come back today and I was very glad to see him and I started a conversation with him. But when the thout about Butch comes to my head I try to chase it away. And saw to myself that that Butch gets on my nerves and I don't think about him and continyeu conversations with my boy friend, my real boy friend not Butch and not yourself. These are happy hollydays. but I will be thrilled to see you if you don't mind you rite the envelope please du not cross out the name of this place where my hotel is. I am getting very brown I hope to be as brown as Butch so when I see him I will be less worried about him. Well Dugie, all my worries will go away sometime.

Lots of love from Sammy.

P.s. I have a feunny thing to tell you about Butch and about some other things. Why does Butch get on my nerves? If my boy friend dosint or my girl friend in New York or the one at the hotel. Why is Butch the only one who dos? Poor me, to have a friend like that, poor me.

(Below is a drawing of Butch and Sammy in which Butch is saying 'I want to kiss you' and Sammy is saying 'No, no' and crying because of Butch.)

P.S. Poor me, oh la la please rite VERRY SOON. Please rite verry VERRY SOON.

Third letter — undated

Dear Dugie,

I am writing you two letters because I mailed the other letter and just remembert that I had a feau more things to tell you and one of the thing that I wanted to tell you is when I worry about my helf from other. Like ther was and still is a man in this hotel who is Dutch and his wife said he is not well and that he fels like pewking some times and he does not look well and one of his eyrs are deff Because he got water in it and I almost crayd that night when his wife said that. I did not almost cray for the sik man I almost crayd for *me* Because I thought that I was going to get sik like this man and then I rember all that you told and then I said to me self I mite die and then I say to my self Nock it off!

It is a hole lot of nonsense thant I am thinking an then every thing went well for good.

From Sammy

I have been swimming a lot and I have lote of fun swimming. (On the outside of the envelope is written: verry troo and I get very worryet about my helf Sammy.)

My Dear Dougie,

I was glad to get your nice letter I could read it very well But your letters are not cleer enuf.

My loose tooth did not come out yet it is in the same spot as it was be for still iching me.

Sometimes when I get leg pains I say to my self oooo ahhh it might Be POLEO coming up and then I say to my self that I shod just lay in the sun and get sunbernt and if it still hurtes me I begin to worry and I say so posing it is POLEO and when I go to America I will haf to see Butch with Creutches on and what would Butch say anyway what would he say? What could we do together if I had poleo? AH that is a trouble ah we will haf to chace that one away. Wont we? By the way I was verry worried and rilly afraid to send A card to Butch—of the grand canion where I was and it was verry nice you know Dougie that this time it is the trouth that I am rilly Be ginning to get afraid of Butch for he just got on my nerves But now I am rilly Begning to worry about Butch and I may not even go to see him.

By the way I sent this card to Butch with frite! I will be going back to new york on the 10 of september and I will there more than a week to see you know WHO! By the way there is a lady in my hotel who has bad armes and she likes to pat people a lot and it exciting me when she does that Because she has Bear armes and pink albos and I wich that I cood feel hur Bear armes.

You know Dougie that with out my hands I would be very sad Because I wouldn't Beable to feel things or toutch. By the way this lady cant wolk well and she has to hold on to the star Bannistor (here follow two completely illegible lines) . . . that's hur trouble not my trouble so I shod not worry about that stuff. I have lots of drems But I will tell you my drems when I get back to Paris. I am having a very nice vachation and a hope that you have too. And that things go well and that you are okey Because I am not Because of that worrying Butch who worres me in fear. My telephone number is . . . . . and my holadays will Be over on the 6th of August and I will be glad to see you. Dont forget about that sik and berd armes wommin. I swimming well. Best witches from Sammy.

PS Tell please all about your vachitoun. And PLEASE WRIT M.O.R.E. if you can. And please write more quike. PLEASE please please.

PS This lady has to hold on to the Bannistor that is what the made says the part that you can't read.

Fifth letter — undated

Dear Dougie,

Your letter was very intersting and it was interstig all that you told me about Spane. As you know now I am less afraid of my fealings about Butch so now I am much less worried. Would you please tell me why my letter before the last one took so long to be posted?

How are your sons and dotors? And how is your husband is he okey? Is your little dog with you?

You know dougie that you did not answer one of my cwechstions about Butch. I asked you what would Butch say IF I HAD POLIO and I had to see him with cruches?

In one of your letters you made a bad mastake about the lady who had one BAD LEG and she had NICE BARE ARMES not Bad Armes. She had a bad leg and that is what I worred about. But I liked her BARE ARMES but sometimes I think how nice it would BEE to pat at her bare armes and LOOK at her pink elbos. She has pink albos. But I dont. I just find that I cant.

Well Dougie I will probabley go to the Bain Deligny where I am swimming and get sunbernt and get my HELF Back.

Love from Sammy.

PS. We will see when you get back which is the helfiest and the braunist of us? I am hafing a lovely time thes days

Butch dos not get on my nervs verry much, Sammy.

(Here follows a drawing which really bears some resemblance to Sammy.) SELFPORTRET.

I make lots of pantings and sketchs. I have drems sometimes. But I will tell you about them back in Paris. (Two illegible lines.)

PS The man with the Baer chest casted a sklptur of a horse that I made. Fur wonce I less worried about his Bear Chest. I am used to the fealings of IT.

(This letter followed me around on holiday so Sammy received a very late reply.)

Sixth letter—undated (Sammy is now back in Paris)

Dear Dougie,

I am very *furiess* Because you havint Been writing me I wrote a nice Long Letter and you did not anser it and if you are not careful I will give you a big soit on your fat bottom now you just wach your self and you better anser my TWO!!!!!!!!!!!!! Letters or els you will get one of thes soits when I see you. Will you stop Being so Frech and not writing. But what is this? That you dont write me attall? Now hirry up and write me with no seen and no complants or els I will get mitie mad after you give your big bottom a Big Soit.

My fealings about Butch are getting much less worrying indeed. And Butch at this momont is getting on my nervs less and less and less. As a matter a fact I feel less afraid of my fealings. I haf written to my psychoanalist in America I like better than you Because she ansers my letters I am *dubbley* mad when you do not write then I am when the outher people do not write to me. Becasue you are my DEAR DOUGIE you are. MY PSYCHOANALIST. You are my own Psychoanalist. MINE!! You belong to me Sammy. You shour do.

I write to my girl friend the one who I was with in Summer Vachation. In case you forgot my address is . . . . And when you write to me have your mail go BY AIRMAIL!!! Pleaze DO.

From Sammy. Dear Sammy.

Good Butch. Sometimes he is good. Oooooo! But not always but Butch is not good when he gets on my nervs.

PS. I had lobster for lunch. But you dident! Write please.

Seventh letter—Saturday morning

Dear Dougie,

If you don't mind I had one of the nervus dreems about Butch S. Jones Jnr. and in the dreem there was a bunch of children and Butch was there and so was a friend of mine who was at my camp too and Butch all of a sudint he kissed me on the chec and I almost fanted Because he kissed Me. and when he kissed me I was rilly saying in my head KEEPON! In the dreem he pated me on the chest with his cold hans and I think that a feau times in the dreem Butch was getting on my nervs. And After that part my Father was in the dreem and he had his Bear Bottom showing. And in a nother part

244

of the dreem my mother was good and nakad and I wanted to pat her Bottom. And my mother sed if you do you will get a soit.

Oh oh it is not troo that Butch is getting less on my nervs I am sorry to say that because of this dreem of mind I am worred and fritend and I mite as well not see him atall dont you think that is a good Idea? I am soffring with frite because of Butch. You know Dougie that I wish that kissing was not INVENTED. I had a nother dreem that I was in a sinagog with MY FATHER. And I was so posed to write a storry of my life not your life and I started to write the Lords Prear but my Father in Law told me to stop and that was all. And a long time ago I dremt that Butch was there and my fingers fell oh and I was in a grate terrer and I cryd when I saw my fingers fall to the ground Because I could no feel things.

Best Love, Sammy.

PS. I will have my own pasport to go to America.

(Here follows a drawing of two boys kissing. One is labelled 'Good Sammy, poor Sammy' and the other 'Bad Butch getting on my nervs.' Underneath this is written 'My fingers mite foll off.')

PS. I am going to the Bain to get my helf back. Sinagog is important to me!!!

PS. PLEASE TELL ME THE THOUT TO MY DREEM
Please Dougie, PLEASE write soon. Comon. Do write soon to Sammy.

PS. I dremt that I had two holes in my ches just like MY Father. Father — Man with the Bad Chest.

Sammy.

Eighth letter — 22 August 1955 (Post card of Champs-Elysées)

Dear Dougie,
I had another dreem about Butch But it was not quite as bad as the fearst one. And in this dreem Butch was fighting people who I do no like. I will hope to see Madame Dupont quite soon and I will be very glad to see her. I love you, Sammy.

. . .

On her return, Sammy's mother told me that although Sammy did not show her the letters he wrote to me, he sometimes let her read my replies. In reading these she had the impression that she understood better what Sammy was going through at that time, and that this had helped both parents at a certain moment to deal with Sammy's difficulties.

Sammy's highly individual letters eloquently express both his feelings and the thinking difficulties against which he was constantly struggling. He is of course extremely anxious about the coming separation of which the summer vacation is but a forerunner. At this time his attachment to Butch is his sole resource, but this displacement in turn awakens guilt and feelings of great danger. In the dream 'where Butch was there and my fingers fell off' he is showing us that he can deal with frightening longings by just cutting off all feeling in a physical sense in the hope of dealing with emotional feeling in this way. 'I cried because I could not feel things.' He does not want to renounce his capacity for feeling. He also longs to feel and to feel for 'the lady with bare arms'; behind both Butch and this lady is the image of his mother. But his love for his mother is also 'sad love'. He can only feel close to her in a sad and distressed way, and added to this there are oedipal anxieties—displaced as we can see on to the hotel-lady's husband, and Sammy's concerns about this man's illness.

155th Session (Tuesday 23.8.55)

Sammy mentions his letters with great shyness. He goes on to talk of a project he has referred to before—of having lunch or dinner with me before he leaves for the States. In the past we have discussed this desire of Sammy's in the light of a flight from the analytic situation. This time he says that he has discussed the matter with his mother and has permission to invite me to dinner at his home, or to invite me to lunch with him at a restaurant. He recalls the analytic implications we have already discussed, then adds significantly, 'But this time Dougie, it's real. I would enjoy having lunch with you, and I will be very well-behaved.' Partly out of countertransference reasons, and partly because I feel that Sammy is making an effort to dissolve his transference attachment, I discuss the preposition on a reality basis, and tell Sammy to thank his mother for the invitation, but that I shall myself invite Sammy to lunch with me, in town, before he leaves. He is delighted with this plan, then sets it aside as

246

something extra-analytic. He talks briefly of Butch but only to say that he is nervous about the coming meeting. He bewails the limited time left before his departure.

He asks if I think his analysis will make more 'progress' if he is in love with me, and adds, 'But I *am* in love with you. Now we'll see how quick it'll go!' When I inquire into the idea that being in love would hasten the analysis he tells me he recently went to see the Danny Kaye film *Knock on Wood* in which the analytic patient falls in love with his female analyst, and they both live happily ever after.

Sammy takes up the theme of his constant concern to eat a lot because of his ever recurrent worries over his health. 'You know, Dougie, I don't overeat just to have fat arms and a fat bottom.' He adds that he also overeats to become bigger than Butch. He draws an arm with a knife stuck through it, and recalls a dream in which he saw a hand with a knife through it. In the dream he 'wanted to have the flesh for himself'.

    S. – I wonder why it's always arms?
J. M. – Why do you think?
    S. – Well, they're good and fat. Well—maybe. I had another dream though, that I was trying to crawl into a hole for safety. I wanted to touch something in there that I wasn't supposed to, and all my fingers dropped off.

He continues spontaneously to talk of his mother and the 'sad and happy love' he had written about in one of his letters. He explains that 'sad love' is when he and his mother have been very angry with each other, and after the quarrel they make it up again. Happy love is without quarrels.

156th Session (Wednesday 24.8.55)

Many Butch fantasies today, but their content is changing. Butch is more often spurned by Sammy who is represented as having the situation well in hand. In one day-dream, Butch dies while Sammy is 'good and alive, and in Butch's place there is only a pile of whitened bones'. Following a day-dream in which Sammy is being pursued by Butch, he brings up the idea that he must find a way of getting back to the peaceful days when he did not know Butch, and there was no one that counted in his life.

247

J. M. – That sounds like a return to the 'stone feeling' instead of real feelings.

S. – Oh no Dougie! That stone feeling has gone for ever and ever. And the dream feeling and the vanishing thoughts! I don't think it'll ever happen again. All all gone.

J. M. – This means that now you can allow yourself to have strong feelings even if they are sometimes sad, or fierce and frightening?

Sammy elaborates a Butch fantasy in which they are friends but rather indifferent to each other. He then admits for the first time that he is not at all certain that Butch ever really kissed him. He remembers that Butch was very kind to him.

S. – Oh but I wish kissing hadn't been invented, then I wouldn't have to have all these frightening ideas about Butch. Now I can see Butch tied to a tree. And I come up and kiss him and kiss him until he suffers just as much as I do.

J. M. – So loving is still connected to attacking and suffering?

S. – Yeah — I don't know why. Oh but it's like that day I wrote to you about the sad love I made with my mother. Dougie, that day I *knew* that my feelings about Butch are all mixed up in my feelings about my mother. But I don't think my mother kissed me too much. I always thought she didn't love me enough.

157th Session (Thursday 25.8.55)

Sammy is in a very gay and happy mood. He asks me several times how I think his worries are going, and says that many of his distressing feelings have gone for good.

S. – But there's some new worries that have taken the place of the old ones. It's a damn shame I always have troubles.

J. M. – Can you tell me something about the new ones?

S. – Well, the biggest trouble is about my health. It's like I have to keep thinking about it or I'll get ill. Then my next trouble is that when I grow up, I'll have to go into the navy, like my father, and get killed. Then there's one more trouble. My father sometimes says things that bother me. One day he told me that he would have to stop me coming here because you didn't tell me that playing with matches in the chimney was dangerous. But one good thing, my worry about Butch isn't very great today. It's a much bigger worry about my father. Now let's talk about our having lunch together, Dougie.

J. M. – Well I'm just wondering if that has something to do with the worry about what your father might think. Perhaps you feel he will be cross about our having lunch together. As though you were going to be like Danny Kaye and his analyst, with me. As though you would like to take mother away from Dad.

Sammy is very displeased by this interpretation, and makes it clear that he wishes in no way to discuss the oedipal anxieties involved. He compares me unfavourably to his New York analyst who ate ice-cream with him and there were no 'thoughts'. Thereupon he says he is going to write a newspaper article about me. He writes the following:

'This young lady is a psychoanalyst. She likes to find out why different people have certain troubles. I'm afraid she did not listen to her teacher who taught her to be a psychoanalyst. In some ways she did, but in the way that she didn't she is not very understanding about different things like my other psychoanalyst was and those things are that she is not so pleasant. But in some ways she is.'

(He breaks off to tell me that I must not analyse the reasons why he wants to take me to lunch, and again refers to the ice-cream given by the former analyst two years ago. He continues the 'article'.)

'Sometimes she takes a long time to help me with these troubles. She is a tiny bit lazy. But anyway she is a fine person to go to after all. And she is quite nice and quite normal. What I mean by normal is that she is sometimes quite smart and uses her nut and knows what she is doing.'

He stops writing to plunge right into a long Butch story, and imagines himself arriving in New York on crutches with his arms broken, and various other forms of mutilation. I tell him he prefers to see himself all damaged rather than face his feelings about Butch. Then, we talk about the whole Butch story being used here rather than thinking about his fear of his father's disapproval, if he loves me or his mummy too much. Without a word Sammy takes up the pencil again and writes:

'This Dougie is very strong in the head, but she is not very soothing.'

249

S. – But I think I would rather know what my troubles are anyway than get them soothed away!

158th Session (Friday 26.8.55)

Sammy tells me that last night the counsellor from the holiday camp where he met Butch, had arrived in Paris, and came to see him. Sammy asked him innumerable questions about Butch in order to compare the reality with his fantasies; for example he learned that it was he who was always running after Butch and not the contrary. The monitor also said that Butch was very much loved by all the boys in the camp, and that he was a good influence on boys who quarrelled and made trouble.

Sammy then decides to write a newspaper story in order to make known the reality concerning Butch. The first chapter attempts a realistic appraisal, but in the second the erotic elements dominate, and Sammy defends himself against this by imagining that he will reject Butch.

Mr Butch S. Jones, Jnr.

This is a great article about Mr Jones jnr, and is to tell you that this young man of 11 years is one of the greatest campers in the U.S.A. This young man is a leader of all the children, I wish that I knew the name of his camp. I have heard that his camp is great and Mr Butch S. Jones is heard of as one of the greatest boys of his age. He is very nice. His counsellor says he calms people down and his friend says that he kisses people and his friend Sammy says that Butch Jones gets on his nerves because this young man kisses him. This young man pats people all the time on their chest like this friend of his dreamed about one night. His friend just can't stand Butch sometimes but he is alright in the end of this great story of Mr Butch Jones who gets on my nerves.

He has such a sweet face and he is very great and full of fun and mischief. He is a mischief-maker—all that boy.

Chapter 2

He likes base-ball a lot and he got very mad sometimes about little things. He is thin and brown—he tells jokes sometimes. I didn't like it when he got mad. We used to pretend to fight, and I always fight my hardest wrestling more or less and he was so kind to me that I was always afraid he would kiss me. I had lots of fun with him but I never used to kiss him. I only kissed him about once or twice. The summer before we didn't know each other and I was much happier. If I was in my flat with all my friends I wouldn't talk to Butch. It made me laugh when my psychoanalyst told me why—she said I was too scared. And now this story ends. Mr Butch S. Jones jnr is the greatest boy for this kissing business.

159th Session (Friday 27.8.55)

Sammy again spends the session making efforts to integrate all the news given by the counsellor into his system of ideas about Butch. He writes another 'newspaper article'.

Story No. 2 of Butch S. Jones Jnr.

Oh that Butch gets on my nerves. He looks down and sees my face and I don't like him—it gets closer and closer but I still don't see him. Then I kiss him. That was awful, isn't it. Butch scares me because he gets mad. It's just because it's against the custom I don't want him to kiss me. Be prepared. Be prepared to hold your liquor like a man. Fight for Harvard's glorious name. Here's the old dope peddler who gives the kids free samples. He knows full well they'll be tomorrow's clientele, with his powdered happiness and all.

Story No. 3 of Mr Butch S. Jones Jnr.

This Butch gets on my nerves because he wrote me a letter this morning. I don't wish to go but to stay with my father. More important than that dope Butch. Big fat dumb old Butch made me break my glasses because he gets me so nervous and excited. It worries me a lot because he says he thinks about me. Even my psychoanalyst doesn't like him 'cos he gets on my nerves. My psychoanalyst gets on my nerves too. Even my father does without my noticing it, but Butch most of all. This is the letter Butch wrote to his friend Sammy.

(Sammy then reads out a friendly boyish letter.)

That what you just heard was a letter from bad evil Butch to nice
Sammy. I should say back to him, 'Your letter was awful. You just
get on my nerves so much. No love, Sammy.'

You know, oh people, it can't keep up this way for 20 years. One
camp summer is exciting but that's enough. That Butch is like an old
milk chocolate because he's so mean to me. He's not so bad but that's
what I mean. I'm such a nice boy, but Butch is afraid of his own
feelings about me. He gets so much on my nerves there's nothing left
to be afraid of. He's the opposite to me. He's got all the bad feelings.
I have what is good and it turns bad in him. He may have got more
healthy than me at camp. If I was still like the days before, I would
sing the Funeral March on him. He can go to hell!

160th Session (Monday 29.8.55)

Sammy announces that his father's car was stolen during the week-
end. So far the police have found no trace of it. He adds that it is too
bad, because he is of the opinion that my husband stole it. Although
he laughs at this idea as improbable he nevertheless remains rather
agitated. He begins to write a letter to Butch, a real one this time,
which announces his date of arrival, flight times, etc. The letter is
strictly factual, rather dull and in marked contrast to the vivacity of
the pretended letters. He jumps up without warning and for the first
time in a long while slaps me on the arm, saying that it's a bad thing
that his father's car has been stolen.

J. M. – The fact that your father's car has been stolen seems to make
you afraid that he has lost some of his power and that I have
taken it away. You feel less strong because his car is lost and
that makes you cross with me.

S. – Yes, it's your fault! I'm going to punch you in the belly.

He becomes very aggressive and makes threatening gestures towards me. I interpret his upset as being allied to the idea that his
father's car represents something masculine and valuable like a penis
and it's as though he thinks I have it in my belly.

S. – Oh that makes me think of a dream I had last night! I had a
long crack in the skin of my hand, but I was frightened to
touch it. I blew the edges apart and it opened up wide. Then
I put my hand in and rubbed the inside.

Sammy adds that he often thinks he would like to touch the organs inside his body. Following the imagery of the dream we talk about his liking to get pleasure out of touching his penis and the frightening ideas that come in at the same time. Sammy says he feels happier about his penis these days and seemed to suggest that his anal interests have given way to phallic ones. The session is dominated, however, by the deeper anxiety that the things inside him are threatened by me. I am abandoning him, thus making it impossible for him to retrieve all that he fears I have taken from him.

He then writes a letter to his New York psychoanalyst telling her he loves her better than me and that he will be seeing her soon. He puts the letter on the table saying I can post it if I want to, but that he won't give me the address.

161st Session (Wednesday 31.8.55)

Sammy makes a drawing of me, defending him against Butch, followed by a drawing of 'Butch's analyst' being very cross with Butch. He then imagines a play-scene, and writes down the dialogue as follows:

Sammy – I wish that Butch didn't kiss me all the time.
Analyst – Ah ah you don't have to worry. Butch is getting very badly punished by his psychoanalyst. Just tell your troubles and we'll go out and have an ice-cream together.
Sammy – It takes one to know one. Joke.

Psychoanalyst laughs ha ha ha and pats Sammy on the back. Both laugh ha ha ha . . .

Butch – Lucky Sammy to have such a nice psychoanalyst. I just can't stop kissing Sammy. I like his cheeks and he's my friend. I like to pat him because he's cute.
Analyst – Now you shouldn't kiss him. It's against the custom! If I catch you doing it any more you'll get *slapped*!! Sammy's nice but you're bad!!!

She slaps him hard because Butch says they must kiss. And that is the end of Butch's kissing for good.

Sammy – Ha ha Butch ha ha.

Sammy then begins a letter which starts 'Dear Kisser' but it doesn't progress further than that. He continues to talk about ways of escaping from the Butch situation although his anxiety seems markedly lessened. He uses me here as a protective superego figure for both himself and Butch. This is also used as a defence against my 'rejection' of him.

162nd Session (Friday 2.9.55)

Sammy brings a dream. He is peeping through the shutters of a house where he can see a lady with bare arms. He goes on to talk of the shutters of his grandfather's house, of the death of his grandfather and his wish to peep on him. He also talks of wanting to peep in on his mother. He has always wanted to know what she is doing when she is in a room with the door closed. Immediately afterwards he refers again to the theft of the car, and hits me. He then asks if I am afraid of smacking myself and what would I do if my son were to hit me.

J. M. – Perhaps you're thinking of things you would do with your mother in the room with the closed door.

S. – You're very smart Dougie!

He goes on to talk about the hotel lady and how he day-dreamed that she was holding him and rubbing her bare arms against him. He would look up under her armpits and had fantasies of attacking them with pencils and needles. He then makes a drawing of Butch spying on him, followed by a number of others depicting the coming meeting with Butch. He finishes by writing a 'letter' to Butch in which he tells him not to be afraid.

163rd Session (Monday 5.9.55)

The session is full of exciting fantasy, stimulated in Sammy by the fact that I am wearing a summer frock with short sleeves. He goes on to elaborate yesterday's bare-arm fantasies.

1. He wants to hit women's arms until they bleed and wants to tear the flesh from the bones, 'but thoughts don't help me, it's only action that helps'.
2. He wants to suck and bite my armpit until 'white blood comes out'.

3. He would like to run a knife through my arms.

While outlining these ideas he intersperses remarks such as 'don't bite me', 'don't hit me' and squeals with excitement. I show him that the biting, hitting ideas are presented as an exciting game for two people. He immediately jumps to talking about Butch, imagining that he is in bed, his leg temporarily paralysed 'and Butch is acting as my baby-sitter'.

J. M. – So in this day-dream Butch is taking the place of your mother?

This leads to a drawing of himself and Butch as siamese twins who are later cut apart. (Fig. 8.) Butch wears a broad smile whereas Sammy's mouth is non-smiling.

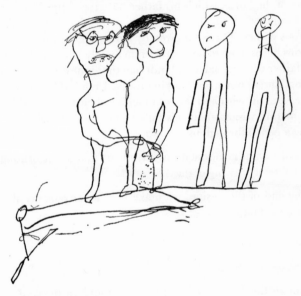

FIG. 8

J. M. – Once again you're joined to Butch like a baby might be with its mother. Maybe you feel about Butch as though he were the other half of yourself?

Sammy makes another series of drawings in which Butch is punished in various violent ways. He is reduced to raw bits of steak, squashed between doors, etc. The last drawing is a portrait of Sammy

255

who has been sleeping and who wakes up to discover that all his ideas about Butch are only a dream. He has no friend!

Sammy comes back to angry day-dreams about me. He would like to run a pencil through my palate, but adds that he wouldn't do this if I were his real mother.

J. M. – So I'm a bad person to whom you can do these things, and then you need do only nice, happy things with your mother?

He draws from memory a tethered horse taken from a postcard his father has given him. While talking of 'beautiful postcards of prehistoric animals' he jumps up and says he wants to bite me. I suggest he wants to be like the fierce animals with me, but that the drawing of the horse, which his father has given him, is represented as well-tethered, and that this is a protective idea against his dangerous wishes. This is followed by a drawing of two animals with enormous horns, nose to nose, and immediately afterwards a drawing of 'my father with his palette'. Underneath this he draws a rhinoceros charging, and another one walking away. I remind him of the rhino fantasies and his wish and fear of touching their horns, and link it to his conflicting wishes about his father and about Butch, and about running a pencil through my 'palate'.

S. – All I want is to touch my own heart and feel it beating! (He makes a drawing of this.)

At the end of the session, we make final arrangements about the luncheon next day.

Lunch (Tuesday 6.9.55)

Although this has not often been mentioned in the session notes, Sammy frequently spoke of having lunch with me before his departure. He insisted that this should not take place immediately before his departure, but a few days before his last session, so that we could talk about it. I give Sammy the choice among several restaurants, and he chooses a Japanese one. He asks that we should first go for a walk. During this walk Sammy tries to embarrass me by silly behaviour (as he does with his mother), such as standing under a fountain until he is soaked through! He was very animated, and full of questions the rest of the time.

Once at the restaurant, he behaves quite appropriately, displays considerable charm to the waiter, shows an interest in the menu and the choice of dishes. He asks the waitress to explain the Japanese letters to him. Eats enormously and with great enjoyment, then asks if we can visit the Sacré-Coeur (where he hides hoping to make me think he has fallen from the top). We go to the Place du Tertre for ices and drinks while Sammy relives all that has happened during the day. He makes a great fuss about returning to my house where his mother is waiting to collect him. Once back he tells her he has had a marvellous day and thanks me very much, 'especially for having spent so much money on me'.

Sammy's behaviour on this rather unusual outing is contradictory. Out of doors he behaved rather like a high-spirited three-year-old, but during the luncheon, and at the café in the Place du Tertre, he is interesting, intelligent, and indeed charming.

164th Session (Wednesday 7.9.55)

Sammy goes over every detail of yesterday's outing. He repeats again how happy he was, how he feels 'that it went off so well' and that he didn't feel at all bad or frightened. He goes on to talk about the coming voyage to New York, and says that his father is very excited about it, because the 'plane will have real beds in it. Sammy accuses his father of being babyish for being excited with so little cause. He then tells me that one day he came in and found his father gazing at his own hands. His father told him that he was thinking what wonderful things hands were.

S. – Isn't he silly? I hate my father to be excited like that.
J. M. – I wonder if you're afraid of your father's excitement in the same way as you are of Butch's excited feelings. Perhaps your real worry is to do with your own feelings towards your father. And towards your own hands.
S. – That's as may be, but I prefer you to talk about Butch rather than my father!

He makes a drawing of his father and himself both swimming, followed by a drawing of Butch and himself who are represented as birds flying. Each of them has an island of his own but Sammy has a much bigger island and has also taken a bit off Butch's island. The

257

next drawing shows Butch and Sammy naked in the trees. On one side there is a big house belonging to Sammy and on the other a little bashed in one for Butch. Sammy then jumps up and says he wants to slap my arms. I point out that he can support a fantasy of bare bodies now in connection with Butch, providing he is bigger and stronger, but not with me because of the conflicting feelings that women's bare arms arouse in him. He calms down immediately and makes a drawing 'in the style of Fernand Léger' called 'Big breasts and big fat arms'. The final drawings are a 'close-up' of Butch and a portrait of 'Butch bombed by Sammy who is in a 'plane'. Underneath he writes, 'I am so happy now that Butch is dead'.

165th Session (Thursday 8.9.55)

Sammy draws himself and Butch swimming. Sammy is having lots of fun and Butch is chasing him. It is the second to last session. Fantasies about Butch and conflicts about leaving me make up most of this session. He expresses the idea that finding Butch again will make up a little bit for losing me. He says he will write letters and that I must answer them all.

166th Session (Friday 9.9.55)

S. – Oh Dougie, it's the very last day. What shall we talk about?

He sits quietly for a moment, then makes a drawing which he labels 'Me dead'. When I ask him to talk about this drawing and its depressive feeling he says it doesn't matter, it's just a letter from Butch which has killed him. I interpret this as his feeling of being abandoned by me, and his wish to get letters from me.

S. – I ought to slap you. Oh that Butch, he gets on my nerves.

Then follow three more drawings.
1. Butch who is crying because Sammy is dead. Butch is holding Sammy in his arms. (Fig. 9.)
2. Butch is kissing Sammy who is still dead.
3. Sammy is dead and in heaven and Butch is praying for him.

It is the end of the session and I tell Sammy we have no more time now. He stands for a long time in the doorway looking at me wistfully.

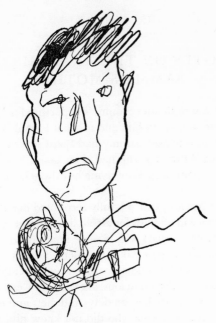

FIG. 9

S. – Oh Dougie, Dougie. Is our time up?

Looking a little bewildered he turns to go then runs back suddenly into the room.

S. – Dougie I'll be back. I'll be back to see you one day.

. . .

Sammy left for New York the following day. Thus his analysis after only eight months' treatment, still in its beginnings, came to an abrupt end.

NOTES ON THE ANALYSIS OF
SAMMY'S MOTHER

In November, a month after Sammy's departure for New York, Mrs Y telephoned to talk about him and to ask if I would consider taking her into analysis. She said Sammy had spent several happy days in New York with Butch and she had then taken him to the Special School. He had wanted to write to me but the school finally decided against this.

At our first interview, which is fully recounted here, Mrs Y told me she had been twice in analysis for alcoholism, two years with a female analyst and later two years with a male analyst. On both occasions she had felt forced to undertake treatment, first by her doctor and then by her husband. This time it was her own decision. Her reasons for choosing me, to her conscious knowledge, were that she felt I would understand both her anxiety and her ambivalence about Sammy better than someone who did not know him and, secondly, Sammy had once said, 'My New York analyst was in love with me but Dougie really likes me and that's even better.' Mrs Y decided there and then that she would come to see me one day. We were able to understand later that this meant I would not take Sammy away from her and would indeed grant her the right to have a son and to love him. She was also reassured that I would not love her too much. Loving relationships frightened her as much as they did Sammy.

Mrs Y felt an urgent need to talk about Sammy. Since leaving him in the United States she grieved for him and also showed considerable mistrust of the Special School. It was her opinion that the Director wished her to give up her son completely and that he regarded her too as psychotic. Her already intense guilt feelings about Sammy had increased. She wondered whether her alcoholism was responsible for Sammy's disturbed state, and now doubted her ability to be a good mother to her small daughter. She went on to talk about her sexual difficulties and in particular her diminishing sexual desire. Her pathological drinking seemed to occur as a means of avoiding acute social anxiety when she was alone. She felt that her four years of analysis had brought little change but that this was in large part due to her acute anxiety at having to lie on the couch where she could not see the analyst. In order to control this situation she had prepared her sessions in advance, and talked without stopping but also without ever saying the things that worried her most. We decided that she would sit up during the present treatment, which began a fortnight later on a four-times-a-week basis. The analysis lasted barely a year, with prolonged interruptions due mainly to holidays. There were eighty-four sessions in all.

Of this fragment of analysis I shall report only those facets which might enrich our understanding of young Sammy and in particular of what he represented unconsciously for his mother. There was a predominance of oral-phallic drama in Mrs Y's fantasy life, as there was in Sammy's, and her ego structure was also very fragile although not dominated by psychotic mechanisms. In her first sessions, when she was not talking of her husband and their disagreements, she talked mainly about her mother. 'My mother was beautiful and accomplished, far beyond anything I could hope to be—or so I thought—but she was extremely cruel. In her frequent rages she would beat me unmercifully. We were all frightened of her at those times, even my father. I remember once that he and my two brothers stood watching while she beat me very severely and none of them dared to move to help me. . . . I could do nothing without mother's help and if she were not with me or watching over me I would feel panic-stricken. She encouraged me to act on the stage, but she was the only person in the audience who counted. She made me go horse-riding, but if she did not stay with me I became terrified. She even wrote all my first love letters for me. . . . The first time I had to go to a dance I was allowed a whisky to supply the courage to go alone without mother. . . . Since she had once suffered from encephalitis she was always tired and she made my brother and me sleep for several hours every afternoon. We were so terrified of waking her we didn't move even to urinate . . . she died when I was seventeen.'

But even after her death, alcoholic drinking continued to give Mrs Y 'the courage to go alone without mother' except that now she and her father would go out drinking together until her father remarried two years later. Then Mrs Y would drink with friends—or drink alone.

After several love relationships with men who frightened her (largely because of the panic aroused by her own fear of sexual excitement) she met Karl Y and married him in her early twenties. 'I told you how I never knew what I felt about a man if he excited me sexually. With Karl it was different. He did not attract me in this way but he made me feel safe. He would get very angry with me when I did silly things in public and has always been extremely anxious about my over-drinking. . . . Sometimes he treats me like a little girl.' It became clear through the transference relationship (in which Mrs Y wanted the analyst to behave towards her in the same way as her husband, that is, keep a rigid control over her and her impulses) that she had repeated with her husband the feelings and the situation she had originally known with her own mother.

With the intensification of this form of the mother-transference in the first weeks of her analysis Mrs Y reacted somatically. First she had an outbreak of hives all down the right side of her face. She herself pointed out that it was the side which faced me during the sessions. The next week she had a skin outbreak on her right arm and hand and then some pathology of her right foot (which eventually necessitated a minor surgical intervention). As we began to decode this cryptic body language Mrs Y became deaf in her right ear! This deafness persisted for several days before giving way to dreams and fantasies with frank homosexual content. In the 35th session Mrs Y brought the following dream:

'I am sitting on the floor with a woman and we are both naked. We are adults but we have hairless genitals like children. The woman masturbates me with her foot and I have an orgasm. I put my right foot out to do the same for her and then wake up.' She adds, 'I am hideously embarrassed about this dream because the woman and I are sitting in exactly the same positions as you and I are here.' Associated with this period of her analysis were many fantasies of women felt to possess unusual attributes and with whom Mrs Y believed it was hopeless to compete. In analysing this idealised transference material she began to realise how much deprivation and suffering she had felt in relation to her own mother, whom she had also idealised to the detriment of her own narcissistic image. These conscious fantasies were accompanied by many dreams of oral incorporation of which the two following are typical: 'I dreamed I was with you and you offered me some very special white fluffy bread just like I used to buy in the States. I put it in my basket but it immediately disappeared leaving just an empty space.' (Her oral love leads only to further loss and loneliness; nothing good can be retained.) In this same session she brought a second dream. 'I am staring at an English setter. Oh I'm sure that's you. You're English and all you do is sit! Anyway, then two men are walking along with this dog and they are cutting it up and eating chunks of it. I try to join them but they push me away.' (Once again she is left with nothing. The bad-dog-woman is the sexual woman, the one gets eaten by the men and the little girl gets none of her. In her better aspects she is good food, fluffy white bread, but this too leaves only emptiness and is in any case lacking in substance.) We were able to see the extent to which Mrs Y's libidinal energy was directed to maintaining an oral and masochistic relation to the mother image from whom she felt incapable of detaching herself. Her intense eroticisation of this relationship with the dead mother was now transferred to Sammy. She attempted to reproduce with him the same kind of painful relationship in which sadomasochistic and oral elements predominated. Her almost symbiotic relationship to her own mother had prevented her from developing a true feminine identification with her, leaving a damaged and empty image of herself. Sammy was destined to be the lost object who would fill this frightening gap. To understand how Sammy came to represent also a forbidden object (the father's baby, the phallus which she could not hold and enjoy without incurring the intense anger of the maternal imago) we must first examine Mrs Y's voyeuristic problems and the phallic significance of her oral-incorporative desires.

Due to the decision that Mrs Y should sit up in the present treatment we were able to re-create in the transference the situation of childhood, which brought to light Mrs Y's deep conviction that once out of her mother's field of vision she was in danger. This psychic reality was an important element in her drinking in which she tried rather desperately to recuperate narcissistically a lost object, the mother, the breast and also in her sexual fantasies in which voyeuristic-exhibitionistic drives played a leading role. This need for narcissistic completion and the voyeuristic desire were fundamental elements in the relationship between Sammy and his mother. The voyeuristic element, whose oral character does not need emphasis, was usually tinged with oedipal guilt, but its dynamic roots lay in the relationship with the mother. A typical masturbation fantasy had been that of offering her former male analyst twice the normal fee if Mrs Y could be allowed to masturbate in front of him (she had felt too guilty about these day-dreams to discuss them with him) but now it became possible to interpret these voyeurist-exhibitionist components as a way of keeping forbidden drives at a distance and thus achieve a guilt free contact with the forbidden object by simply looking and being looked at. This brought in its wake a realisation of the aggressive component of Mrs Y's erotic life (against which her voyeuristic defences had, until now, protected her) and she began to understand how closely interwoven were her aggressive and erotic feelings. The following dream which came several sessions after the ones just quoted is evocative: 'I am waiting to see two women whom I hear are very beautiful. They come in wearing thick black veils and they lie down and expose their genitals. One is very hairy but the other is more like a little girl. I ask myself how men can possibly find such a sight beautiful. Then in comes my husband. He offers me a dog biscuit which he holds between his legs. I jump up, catch the biscuit with my mouth and swallow it as though I were a dog.' (The 'sexual-dog-woman' once again.) In her spontaneous associations to this dream Mrs Y recounts a joke. 'A girl is eating cherries in a bar. She sucks each one slowly and sensually while a fascinated man-friend watches her. Suddenly she snaps at one cherry with her teeth. Her friend starts up with a cry and grabs at his penis.' At the end of the session Mrs Y recounted that Sammy had sent his father a cake for his birthday. The night before this dream she and her husband had eaten the cake. She had thought to herself that it was like 'restoring Sammy inside her in some way', but this fantasy did nothing to mitigate her feeling of loneliness and emptiness without him. We see that the dream begins with a search for feminine identification by the the little girl with her mother, but this cannot be accepted, partly because it leads to an aggressive oral incorporative wish in an attempt to achieve some kind of unity. After the story of the girl and the cherries Mrs Y had gone on to recall her tremendous guilt feelings in relation to her mother and in particular an accusation of stealing from the mother. In other words she was guilty of desiring to steal (eat) the penis which belonged exclusively to the mother (as well as her baby boy to whom she felt she had no right either). The girl-and-the-cherries was only one of the many colourful examples that led us to understand that drinking meant also to eat up (and lose) the penis. Her desire was to incorporate and possess its goodness and thus feel fulfilled like a baby at the breast. I remarked that when she described her drinking it was as though she had a penis inside her with good and protective qualities, whereas when she stopped drinking she felt utterly empty. 'That's funny,' she said. 'When I'm hungry I often feel it's my vagina that is empty. I never know whether I want food or sex.' Behind her dream-wish to swallow her husband's biscuit-penis and her conscious association to 'eating' Sammy, Mrs Y expressed a primal scene fantasy founded on her own desire for her mother's breast. Mrs Y's dream life and associations revealed many breast-penis equivalents. These few excerpts will I hope give some idea of the intricately interwoven pattern of desire and oral fantasy in her sessions and the way in which they strikingly resembled Sammy's *conscious* fantasy-life.

I shall now try to present my understanding of what Sammy meant to his mother. If Sammy was a phallic object for his mother (which tended to exclude, for both, the relationship with the father) Sammy's image of himself was deeply interwoven with his mother's oral fantasies. His desperate and uncontrolled impulses to play out his mother's unconscious desires forced her in return to keep him at a distance. 'I never knew what I felt for a man who attracted me and it was much the same with Sammy just as though he aroused me sexually. This made me even more irritated and distant with him. I have the impression that Sammy sensed all of this.' Mrs Y felt these projected feelings existed from the time Sammy was born, and this interfered in her sensuous contact with him at this crucial time. She was afraid to express normal maternal love and tenderness. Later she was surprised and frightened by her intensely aggressive feelings towards him, but in these moments of great anger she would begin at last to feel close to him. 'It was just like those terrible beatings my mother gave me. I think she gave them as much from passion as from anger. I would feel relaxed afterwards. The same thing happened when I hit Sammy. Afterwards we would both be crying and we would cuddle.' I understood for the first time that when Sammy 'was making sad and happy love' with his mother he was actually re-living with her a situation of unfulfilled desire attached to her own childhood.

As the analysis progressed we were able to reconstruct Mrs Y's fantasy attempt to be the phallic completion of her mother, and her subsequent attempt to make Sammy the phallus for which she was searching in her desperate desire to recover her 'whole' self. (One aspect of her compulsive drinking was this same attempt to become whole and to that extent in her imagination she was *protecting* Sammy from the role she unconsciously wished him to play, when she over-drank.) In the 73rd session Mrs Y talked of her depressed feelings following Sammy's birth and she was able to express the idea that this birth was really like a vital *loss*. That night, after the session, she dreamed 'I was in a sort of cot and beside me is a man who at one moment is my brother and at another he becomes my husband. The doctor is about to arrive any moment and I realise I must have an orgasm before he gets here. When he does come it's as though we share some secret. He is very sympathetic.' The room in which the dream is set leads her to remember the room she shared with her brother during the long hours of forced siesta. She then brings memories of a little 'doll-pillow' she had kept throughout her childhood. 'I kept it for years, I always slept with it between my knees and used to masturbate with it. That's when I used to imagine I was being beaten or that I was being exposed to strange and ugly people who were watching me masturbate. This was in the afternoons. Then one day, when I was nine, my mother came in and caught me. And she threw it away. Oh now I think of it, that cot in the dream isn't the bed I had as a child, it's the one I had in the maternity hospital *when Sammy was born*. My husband was there during the delivery. But it was my brother who watched when mother grabbed away my doll-pillow when I was only nine!!' Thus Sammy had become the little doll-pillow which her mother had taken away. An object of guilt-laden desire and forbidden by the mother, Sammy *had to be rejected*. There is a tragic feeling of destiny in the coincidence that Sammy too was 'taken away' from her when *he* reached the age of nine. Equally tragic was her unconscious conviction that orgastic fulfilment could only be hers 'before the doctor came', that is before her mother forbade for ever both the orgasm and the phallic completion which the doll-pillow represented, and which later her baby came to incarnate. However, to the extent to which her associations led her to identify me as the doctor she revealed her hopes that in spite of the fears at the beginning of the analysis that I too would take away her baby and her sexuality, she could now share a secret, the secret of her feminine desires with the 'sympathetic' doctor, as she did in the dream.

The many excitements which Mrs Y sought in alcohol made already a formidable list. Besides being good food and a good mother, a protection against devouring the biscuit-penis and against using Sammy as an object of sexual gratification it became clear that her drinking was finally a proof of her 'innocence'. She was not a rival with her mother for the penis or the baby, but herself a small baby seeking only oral satisfactions. But she had unconsciously stimulated Sammy into playing a role in her voyeuristic fantasies.

These represented a special mode of contact with her own mother. When it was the *mother* who kept the young girl in her field of vision she was able to feel that she really existed. When on the other hand it was Mrs Y who did the looking it became eroticised and thus a way of controlling, and finally outwitting the mother. In the last weeks of her fragment of analysis with me she recounted the following dream: 'I see Sammy wearing an enormous feather hat. He is leaning forward peeping through a venetian blind. Funny I've seen that hat before. Oh yes, in my mother's marriage photo. And those are the same blinds through which I couldn't see anything! The agonies I used to go through over closed doors! My mother blocked up all the keyholes . . . when she was watching me I used to feel immobilised as though I were hypnotised.' In point of fact Mrs Y wanted to watch and to control (hypnotise) her mother—and me, in the analytic situation. It may be remembered that Sammy had an almost identical 'peeping' dream towards the end of his therapy with me. Everything points to the fact that Mrs Y re-lived through Sammy her own voyeurist wishes forbidden by her own mother. Sammy was to express *her* wishes and thus re-create by proxy another link in her primitive bond to her own mother. Her feelings about him were bound to be contradictory. At times she felt him to be a lost object which had therefore to be decathected and kept at the farthest possible distance and at other times he was the forbidden object which she could recuperate in a sado-masochistic, eroticised relationship. Thus she was afraid that her drinking had made him ill; at the same time she felt she had to drink in order to escape the anxiety aroused by a too close relationship with him. By his very illness Sammy was truly hers yet he constantly escaped her.

After the summer holidays Mrs Y reported that she had for the first time in years passed the holidays without any over-drinking, that she had really enjoyed herself and that the old boredom seemed to have disappeared. As she was to leave in a short while to return to the States she wanted to try the last two months without analysis. In the last two sessions we had, after her holidays, she seemed much calmer and she looked much better physically. Her sexual problems on the contrary were only slightly modified, and to some extent I felt that her drinking had been replaced by a rather aggressive relationship with her husband. She kept in touch with me from time to time, and up to her return to the States in January, her former alcoholism did not return.

REPORT FROM THE SPECIAL SCHOOL

Report on Sammy Y (April 1958)

NEARING the end of Sammy's second year with us he said, 'The first year here is to get comfortable, the second year to get acquainted, and the third to get to work.' This seems to have summed up Sammy's stay with us so far.

His first year he experimented in learning how to play with toys and games. Previous to this, with the exception of stuffed animals or art materials, he spent most of his time seeking out adult activities, pretending to an over-sophisticated interest in *avant-garde* paintings, esoteric music and such things, in which he was like an empty copy of his father. His appearance was that of a tired old man, resigned to his fate of being without emotional energy. He used his intellectual precocity to ward off, annoy and provoke us with a continuous barrage of questions which, when answered, only led to endless streams of new questions, and with baiting remarks to the adults who took care of him. He would frequently propose marriage or make sexual advances to counsellors of both sexes, particularly when he was anxious or angry with them.

For some time he was actively involved with one other rather delinquent boy in building elaborate fantasy games, often of a thinly disguised homosexual nature. They would crash cars together, chant together at their counsellors and spin tops in magical ways. Unless firmly controlled, he would become extremely frightened by his many hostile fantasies. Although this served mainly as a discharge for him, it also permitted us slowly to involve him in the use of toys and play more suitable to his age.

For months he made clay 'monsters' which he told stories about and had them give birth to many little babies. These monsters were all characterised by large devouring mouths and long smooth bodies. He began to talk about animals and often played with his favourite stuffed ones during the day. He would ask his counsellor what she would do 'if a lion, tiger and a bear came after you and woke you up in the night'. He began to knock on her door several times during each night and could then talk more and more openly with her about his night fears. As a result of this he became able to fall asleep more gradually and more easily. He now gets a good night's rest most of the time.

Although Sammy has been preoccupied with his sexual fantasies all along, it took a long time before his anxieties about his own sex organs began to emerge. He expressed first in pictures his desire to be both boy and girl and began to use drawings as a means of telling this to us. With some of these pictures went elaborate stories, often of violence to his counsellor or himself when he was angry at her.

Throughout his life Sammy has been riddled with psychosomatic complaints and anxieties about everyday colds and aches and pains. At first he tested us how well we would take care of him and constantly accused us of not getting him medicine, or some magical cure-all. This has changed to an open expression of how worried he is about his body and now shows considerable affect in this area.

He has a greater grip on reality here and seems more motivated to do something about this aspect of his life than any other; this is in part due to his feeling that he cannot yet manage life with his parents. His co-ordination is still somewhat poor, but he can get by in most situations.

At this moment Sammy often looks like a handicapped girl. His voice is effeminate and whispering, and his health a source of constant worry, although he is in excellent physical condition except for being slightly underweight. His facial expressions show a greater depth of sadness, instead of the blank or manic elation with which he came to us. He spends a great deal of time reading on his bed.

Immediately previous to a visit with his parents at Christmas time he continuously tested out who was in control. He went through many elaborate attempts to control his counsellors and in many ways tried to live his life through them, much as his father still tries to do with him. This culminated in an attempt to set fire to a toilet during his visit home, which frightened him very much; mostly because his parents took such an expression of deep hostility so lightly. He was very relieved that we felt it was serious, although we would not punish him for it as he wanted us to do.

In the last few months Sammy has, for him, been rather quiet. It is as if he is slowly developing something that he is not quite sure about yet. He has begun to raise potted plants and takes excellent care of them. It is very important to him to observe how well they grow and he seems to have more confidence in his own future.

In January 1957 we felt that Sammy was ready to be placed in a classroom which emphasises learning through projects and activity, rather than a formal, academic programme. At that time it was our conviction that continued academic acceleration was a drain on his then limited emotional resources.

Understandably, Sammy reacted to this change with concern about his achievement. At first, Sammy remained aloof from the other children. After a few months his growing interest in what was going on in the classroom was manifested in several ways. He watched what other children were doing and listened to what they said. He asked questions about events in their daily life in the dormitory and at times initiated play with them. After a period of becoming acquainted with his teacher and the other children, he availed himself, to some degree, of more childish play and activity. For example, he spent many hours working with clay and building with blocks. He especially enjoyed helping to prepare simple snacks for himself and the other children.

Music appeals to him very much, but now on a more childish level. For several months now he has delighted participating in a rhythm band, and it was a pleasure to watch him enjoy childish games and songs.

Sammy is now doing regular lessons for two or three hours daily. He is usually interested in what he is doing and rarely expresses dissatisfaction about his achievement; this is in great contrast to the past. He is becoming increasingly responsive towards his teacher and is becoming more interested in discussions pertinent to life in the classroom as well as his own concerns.

When Sammy is distressed, particularly for weeks after he has spent some time with his father, he becomes withdrawn and looks sad. His movements are then listless and restricted. In a conflictual situation with another youngster, Sammy usually turns to his teacher with a petulant request that she 'do something'. But it is encouraging that he no longer needs to maintain a negativistic and hostile attitude towards everyone and everything when he is feeling troubled.

Sammy began having individual psychotherapy sessions twice a week with our psychiatric social worker at the end of November 1956. He met this new situation with eagerness. His need to control and ask incessant questions became more marked for a while until he began to trust this new person in his life. He made many attempts to make the individual work fit a pattern he was familiar with and he was quite puzzled when he couldn't get her co-operation. For a while he permitted himself to play, first by making a huge clay alligator, then a large egg that would 'take a year to hatch'. With the clay he was able to be aggressive and eventually with toys too. Play with dolls was spurious and with much hostile behaviour towards the mother and father figures.

The play activities ceased five months after he started the sessions, perhaps because he felt safe enough to talk about what was uppermost in his mind—his own sexual development. He devised a unique way to test out his worker's attitude towards sex by making up all kinds of stories about penises such as 'How the men lost their penises'. This theme had many and varied elaborations. Two months later he made a picture of a blossoming plant. He indicated pleasure by placing notes of music around it and wrote 'Growth' alongside it.

Recently he began talking about his masturbation fears. He used the device of drawing for communicating his worries. Some of these pictures were elaborate and others were simple drawings of how he saw his genitals. He drew a plant he called the 'Yeus' plant which grew in the distant land of South America. It had a red line running through it and it could spit its poison out on women. He said it was a very pretty plant. It had big leaves that could eat people. It needed very little water because it could store water in its big leaves.

In the following week Sammy began talking about his night fears. This time he told a story of the kidnapping of a nude woman. From this time on, for about four months, the theme was nude women and stories and pictures of nude women; he recalled an incident that happened one vacation when he was six. His mother and he were at a resort; his father was not there. His mother had gone to the hotel bar for a drink and later was followed to her room by an intoxicated man. Sammy observed the struggle between his mother and the man in bed and later his mother coming to him in his bed. In talking about this, drawing pictures of the scene, he remembered he has woven this memory in and out of many stories. He was relieved to know that his mother had told us about this when we interviewed her.[1]

At the present time, Sammy has developed a number of psychosomatic complaints—pains in his legs, side and throat. He became intensely interested in three diseases—polio, appendicitis and

[1] Sammy had not actually forgotten this incident. He referred to it frequently at home, and at one moment in his analysis with me utilised it as a screen memory to primal scene anxieties. J.M.

271

cerebral palsy. He has also brought out his anxiety about mental illness by drawing pictures of a woman who developed hydrophobia. He explained that his fear of illness either physical or mental was due to his being worried about his thinness and smallness and to be afraid of hiding his worries. This later was also associated with masturbation which has increased when he discovered that he was developing sexually.

Mr Y spent three months in Paris at the beginning of this year. Sammy became anxious, imagining that his father would marry another woman and that his mother could not be trusted alone. However, he was able to talk about these concerns immediately. He was obviously relieved when his father returned home.

Sammy still has a strong need to test out his worker when he has something new to talk about, but there is far less hostility shown in the testing. It is as though this is a pattern he can't quite give up yet, but the feeling for it is no longer there. He is still afraid that the people in his life are jealous of each other, but again this is less intensified than formerly.

INTERVIEW WITH SAMMY'S FATHER

May 1958

ADMITTING he is rather biased, Mr Y expressed disappointment in the Special School. He finds little change in Sammy despite the reassurances of the Director. While there is gradual progress in school work, Mr Y feels that this was well under way when Sammy left Paris. On the emotional side he feels the progress is nil. Sammy still avoids playing with other children and is solitary and sad. He has no idea how to behave in social situations. Recently his father took him to buy an article of clothing. Sammy would make no choice until he had seen every example of this article to be found in the shop. At home he is provocative and teasing and he demands the constant attention of the adults around him. He is still quite incapable of leading a normal life like other children of his age.

Mr Y then went on to the good aspects of Sammy's current behaviour. He makes obvious efforts to check his endless demands for things and sometimes he even shows genuine pleasure in what is done for him. He recently thanked his father for taking him to a show, which is quite new for him. Formerly he criticised everything that was offered to him or done for him. He is kinder and gentler with his little sister and also has a calmer and happier relationship with his mother.

NOTE, MAY 1958

DESPITE Mr Y's disappointment, we see from the school reports that Sammy is learning to control his impulses to some extent, although it apparently does not carry over as yet to the world outside the school. From the reports he remains as anxious as ever about his body. His hypochondriacal complaints, the anxieties over his height and weight and about his genital organs bear witness to this. The content of his fantasies strangely enough seems little changed. One can detect the continued importance of oral cathexes in the fantasy of the plant Yeus. To ejaculate is at the same time to devour and to incorporate.

In his psychotherapy Sammy would appear to be recapitulating some of the steps covered in his fragment of analysis in Paris. It is interesting that he again represents himself as a growing plant as he had done three years ago. Even if the little plant still eats people, it is nevertheless growing.

J. M.